Hair Loss & Replacement

FOR

DUMMIES

Hair Loss &
Replacement
FOR
DUMMIES®

by William R. Rassman, M.D.,
Jae P. Pak, M.D., Eric Schweiger, M.D.,
and Robert M. Bernstein, M.D.

WILEY

Wiley Publishing, Inc.

Hair Loss & Replacement For Dummies®

Published by
Wiley Publishing, Inc.
111 River St.
Hoboken, NJ 07030-5774
www.wiley.com

WILEY

About the Authors

William R. Rassman, M.D. is a professional inventor with more than two dozen issued or pending patents in a wide range of fields including medical devices, computer software, and biotechnology instrumentation. He introduced the modern standards of care for hair transplantation, pioneered follicular unit hair transplantation, follicular unit extraction, and hair transplant repair, publishing these techniques in prestigious medical journals with Dr. Bernstein. He received the Golden Follicle Award for his contributions to the clinical practice of hair restoration. Dr. Rassman has been featured on TV media events such as ABC's *Extreme Makeover* and programs on the Discovery Channel, the BBC, and many others. Throughout his career, Dr. Rassman's goal has been to make a difference, and among his most notable accomplishments is his pioneering work developing and commercializing the intra-aortic pump, today's standard of care heart pump found in almost every cardiac care unit in the world. Today Dr. Rassman's focus is on his hair transplant practice and the balding blog www.baldlingblog.com, now the largest hair loss Web site in the world. You can find out more about his practice at his Web site, www.newhair.com, and by calling 1-800-NewHair.

Jae P. Pak, M.D. graduated from the University of California, Irvine, with a Bachelor of Science degree in Aerospace and Mechanical Engineering. He then took a brief detour with the U.S. Marine Corp Officer Candidate School in Quantico, Virginia, to pursue his love of aviation. As an engineer, he designed fiber optic illuminators and lighting systems that are used all over the world. Some of his engineering work can be seen on the skyline of Las Vegas and stealth ships operated by the U.S. Navy. Eventually Dr. Pak went on to complete his medical training at the Medical College of Virginia. His interest in medicine crossed paths with Dr. William Rassman's interest in engineering in 1997. Since then, the two have been pioneering hair transplant methods, automation, and instrumentation from the initial follicular unit extraction (FUE) techniques and tools to Hair Implanting Pen devices that are routinely used in his practice. He has collaborated on U.S. Patents with Dr. Rassman and has been intimately involved with innovative hair transplant surgical techniques incorporating new technology. Dr. Pak is also an avid artist and painter, which serves him well in the aesthetics of hair restoration. Dr. Pak continues to develop new surgical techniques and invent surgical instrumentation to further advance the field of hair transplant surgery with Dr. Rassman at the New Hair Institute in Los Angeles.

Eric Schweiger, M.D. is Clinical Instructor of Dermatology at the Mount Sinai Medical Center in New York City. He practices cosmetic and general dermatology with a particular focus on hair loss and its treatment. Dr. Schweiger has served as the primary investigator in clinical research studies involving lasers and light-based treatment, and he has authored numerous articles in peer-reviewed medical journals. Dr. Schweiger received his undergraduate degree from the University of Michigan and his doctor of medicine from the Albert Einstein College of Medicine in New York . He completed his internship in internal medicine at NYU Medical Center and his dermatology residency at the University of Kansas. You can find out more about his practice at www.bernsteinmedical.com.

Robert M. Bernstein, M.D. is Clinical Professor of Dermatology at the College of Physicians and Surgeons, Columbia University in New York. He's recognized worldwide for his pioneering work in follicular unit hair transplantation, follicular unit extraction, and hair transplant repair. Dr. Bernstein has been chosen as one of *New York Magazine*'s "Best Doctors in New York" for eight consecutive years, and he's a recipient of the Platinum Follicle Award for his achievements in surgical hair restoration. Dr. Bernstein has been featured on *Good Morning America,* the *Today* show, and the Discovery Channel. He has appeared on *The Early Show, CBS News,* Fox News, National Public Radio, and in *GQ Magazine, Men's Health,* and *Vogue.* Dr. Bernstein's Center for Hair Restoration in Manhattan is devoted to the treatment of hair loss using pioneering state-of-the-art hair transplant techniques. You can find out more about his practice at his Web site, www.bernsteinmedical.com, and by calling 212-826-2400.

Authors' Acknowledgments

The authors have written numerous scientific articles and textbook chapters for the medical field, but writing a succinct reference book for a wide audience is a uniquely different challenge and in many ways far more difficult. We could never have accomplished this task without the help of our experienced editors Sharon Perkins and Tracy Brown Collins (who are anything but Dummies). We're very grateful for their professionalism and hard work in bringing this book to press.

As hair transplant surgeons, writing about the technical elements of the surgical process was easier than tackling some of the other subjects that fell outside our area of expertise. We want to thank Douglas Hong, who had the insight to point us in the direction to write this book; Dr. Norman Estrin, for his help in explaining issues related to the FDA as well as hair care; and Bret Katz and David Ahdoot of DD Chemco, for giving us very important insights into the fine nuances of the chemicals and ingredients found in various commercial products.

Although there are many people we can acknowledge who helped educate us in the fields of hair and hair restoration, Dr. Richard Shiell stands out because he freely gave us insights from his decades of experience working through the various hair technologies. Also, there are many staff members who have worked tirelessly with us in surgery as part of our teams, hour after hour and day after day, and we wish to acknowledge them as a group.

We want to thank our patients for the faith they put in us as physicians and surgeons. As we were at the forefront of a new hair transplant paradigm, we were fortunate that many of our patients were able to understand this vision and share in its development. We became partners in their surgical care and in the evolution of this exciting new field of hair restoration.

Publisher's Acknowledgments

We're proud of this book; please send us your comments through our Dummies online registration form located at www.dummies.com/register/.

Some of the people who helped bring this book to market include the following:

Acquisitions, Editorial, and Media Development

Project Editor: Tracy Brown Collins

Acquisitions Editor: Mike Lewis

Senior Copy Editor: Elizabeth Rea

Technical Editor: Dr. Ronald Shapiro

Senior Editorial Manager: Jennifer Ehrlich

Editorial Supervisor and Reprint Editor: Carmen Krikorian

Editorial Assistants: Joe Niesen, David Lutton, Jennette ElNaggar

Cover Photo: © BananaStock

Cartoons: Rich Tennant (www.the5thwave.com)

Composition Services

Project Coordinator: Patrick Redmond

Layout and Graphics: Reuben W. Davis, Melissa K. Jester, Christine Williams

Art Coordinator: Alicia B. South

Special Art: Kathryn Born

Proofreader: Evelyn C. Gibson

Indexer: Potomac Indexing, LLC

Publishing and Editorial for Consumer Dummies

> **Diane Graves Steele,** Vice President and Publisher, Consumer Dummies
>
> **Joyce Pepple,** Acquisitions Director, Consumer Dummies
>
> **Kristin Ferguson-Wagstaffe,** Product Development Director, Consumer Dummies
>
> **Ensley Eikenburg,** Associate Publisher, Travel
>
> **Kelly Regan,** Editorial Director, Travel

Publishing for Technology Dummies

> **Andy Cummings,** Vice President and Publisher, Dummies Technology/General User

Composition Services

> **Gerry Fahey,** Vice President of Production Services
>
> **Debbie Stailey,** Director of Composition Services

Contents at a Glance

Table of Contents

Introduction

● ●

*H*air loss—what's the big deal? Everyone loses their hair eventually, right? No point in worrying about it—or buying a book about it. For that matter, how much is there to say about hair loss anyway? And isn't it rather vain to worry about hair loss when world peace still hasn't been achieved?

While we'd be the last to argue that world peace should take a back seat to your hair loss, we think there's plenty to say about losing your hair—which is why we've written this book. We also think that losing your hair can be a crushing blow to your self-esteem, and can affect your social life, work performance and view of yourself.

The good news is there are things you can do to minimize or prevent hair loss, and ways to obtain a whole new head of hair, if you decide to go that route. It may help you to realize the scope of the hair loss problem by considering the following statistics:

- ✔ Around fifty percent of men suffer from some degree of male pattern baldness by age fifty
- ✔ Around twenty million women have significant hair loss at some point in their lives
- ✔ Millions of men have taken prescription medications to prevent or decrease hair loss
- ✔ Approximately 100,000 men have hair transplants every year

Whether you already have significant hair loss, or are just sizing up the other members of your family and fearing that hair loss is in your future, this book will help you face your concerns and weigh your options in the most practical way possible.

About This Book

The goal of this book is to make you more aware of the options you have if you're suffering from hair loss, and to make you more comfortable pursuing those options. Whether you choose to take medication, buy a hairpiece, or go directly to hair transplantation, we want you to be an educated and confident consumer.

We also want you to understand hair: what it is, why it reacts the way it does to the abuse most of us heap on it, and how best to preserve its appearance.

This book is for you if you're concerned about future hair loss or already in the throes of it, or if you know someone who is. You'll learn more here than you ever wanted to know about diseases that cause hair loss, the medications and over the counter options that promote hair growth, how hair transplants are performed, how to choose a good surgeon, and the way hairpieces are made, if you choose to read the whole book.

On the other hand, if you just need quick info on what to expect after hair transplant, or which medications work best, a quick look in the appropriate chapter will give you that info.

Conventions Used in This Book

Every book follows certain styling rules to make it easier for you to find information. In this book, we put important words that we define in the glossary at the end of the book in *italics*. We also put key words in **bold** type so they stand out and catch your attention.

We place all Web addresses in `monofont` to set them apart. During printing of this book, some of the Web addresses may have broken across two lines of text. If you come across such an address, rest assured that we haven't put in any extra characters (such as hyphens) to indicate the break. When using a broken Web address, type in exactly what you see on the page, pretending that the line break doesn't exist.

This book contains sidebars, which are shaded in gray, that contain interesting or fun information, or personal stories about our experiences in the hair loss field. You don't have to read them to understand the principals of hair loss and replacement, but hopefully you'll enjoy reading them when you have time.

What You're Not to Read

Feel free to skip the copyright material, unless you're the sort who has to read everything. You can also skip sidebars, the gray boxed material that contains mostly personal stories which are immensely interesting (and often amusing) but not essential for your knowledge of hair replacement.

You may also want to skip areas marked with the icon Technical Stuff if technical things aren't your strong suit.

Foolish Assumptions

This book is for everyone concerned about their hair in any way, shape or form—if you want healthier hair, more hair, or replacement hair, this book is for you. More specifically, you should read this book if:

- ✔ You know male pattern baldness runs in your family
- ✔ You already have some hair loss and want to know how to slow or stop it
- ✔ You're thinking about taking medication—prescription or over the counter—to slow hair loss
- ✔ You want to conceal your hair loss as long as you can and do not know how to do this
- ✔ You want to buy a hairpiece but don't know where to start
- ✔ You're considering a hair transplant and need more information

How This Book Is Organized

This book is organized into six parts. Each part addresses different aspects of hair loss and hair replacement. This organization makes it easy to find the topic you're looking for. Here's a quick overview of what you can find in each part.

Part 1: Getting to Know Your Hair

The better you know your hair, the better you'll be able to care for it. This section teaches you all about hair—what it's made from, how it grows, and how best to care for it. This part covers everything from the intimate inner workings of a hair follicle to choosing the right shampoo for your hair.

Part II: The Root of Hair Loss: How and Why It Happens

In this part, we look at all the different reasons for hair loss, with a detailed look at the most common cause of baldness, male pattern baldness. We also examine the many different diseases and health issues that can cause temporary or permanent hair loss.

Part III: Creative Techniques for Concealing Hair Loss

When you're looking to conceal your hair loss, this is the section to read. We describe the temporary methods of hair loss concealment such as sprays, as well as hair systems such as toupees, wigs, extensions and weaves. We also give you a complete course in how hair systems are created, how to tell a good hair systems from a bad one, and how to buy quality when you are shopping for a hair system.

Part IV: Pharmaceutical, Laser, and Topical Therapies

In this part, we look into the medicine cabinet for hair loss remedies. We discuss the prescription medications for hair loss, their benefits and limitations, and also look at over the counter and alternative medicines that claim to slow or prevent hair loss. We also describe the use of laser treatments in stimulating hair growth, and tell you what works—and what to avoid.

Part V: Advanced Hair Loss Solutions

If a hair transplant is in your future, this is the part to read. Not only do we tell you how to find the right surgeon, we also tell you how to avoid the wrong ones. We also give you a detailed look into the operating room, and follow you home to help you through the weeks and months after your transplant.

Part VI: The Part of Tens

Every Dummies books contains a Part of Tens section; these are short, pithy, often humorous chapters dealing with the topic at hand. In the Part of Tens, we look at the FDA and the ways it does—and doesn't—protect you from charlatans in the hair replacement field. We also look at the myths of hair loss, a few reasons why hair transplant may be your best bet in the long run, and ten reasons why non surgical replacement may be better in your case.

Icons Used in This Book

This book draws your attention to different types of information by placing four icons in the margins of the text. These draw your attention to bits of information we consider important in one of the following ways:

When we think something is especially important, we mark it with the Remember icon.

Information marked with the Tips icon enhances or simplifies your life in some way.

Pay attention to Warning icons; the information they contain is essential to maintaining your hair—or your health. If we think the information deserves a Warning icon—make sure your read it—and follow our advice!

This book contains a lot of technical information about your hair; while all the info under the Technical icons is interesting and important from a scientific viewpoint, it's not required reading if you're not interested in a lot of scientific or medical detail about hair loss.

Where to Go from Here

As with all Dummies books, this book is set up so you can go to whatever section interests you, read just that section, and come away with all the info you need. Of course, we hope you'll read the whole book, because we feel it contains valuable info, but don't feel like you have to read it all at once or in any particular order.

If you want to delve deeper into hair replacement issues, we've included an appendix at the end of the book which lists sources for more information, as well as for support groups, if you're the type who likes to join organizations.

Part I
Getting to Know Your Hair

The 5th Wave   By Rich Tennant

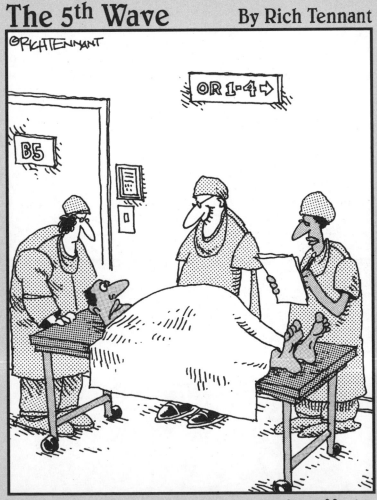

"Included with today's surgery, we're offering a manicure, pedicure, and ear wax flush for just $49.95."

In this part . . .

What is hair, exactly? This part answers all your burning questions about hair: what it's made of, how it grows, and how you should take care of it so that it will last a lifetime — or at least as long your genetic makeup allows it to hang around.

Chapter 1

All About Hair and Hair Loss

· ·

In This Chapter

▶ Getting to know your hair and why you have it

▶ Acknowledging causes and the personal impact of hair loss

▶ Considering temporary and permanent solutions

▶ Looking forward to future developments in the field

· ·

You may wonder how we can write an entire book on the topic of hair loss. You may think hair loss is an incurable condition, so what is there to say about it? But hair loss doesn't have to be inevitable, even if your whole family is balding or thinning. You can take steps to slow hair loss and replace the hair you've lost.

In this chapter, we introduce some facts about hair loss, including who may experience it and, best of all, what your options are when you start to feel air on the top of your head.

Who Cares About Hair? Everyone!

Even people who don't pay much attention to their hair care when it starts to thin or fall out. You may feel somewhat betrayed: You've been kind to your hair, bought expensive shampoos, and kept up with regular maintenance, and this is how it rewards you — by falling out?

We take our youth and our hair for granted as long as we have them. Then, certain things happen as we age — we sag, gain weight, lose muscle tone — and we may not like them, but we know we could fix them by exercise, diet, and lifestyle changes — not that we will, necessarily, but we feel we could if we wanted to. In other words, we still feel like we have control.

And then there's hair. At least every month, in the case of most men, we face our hair in the mirror at the hair salon, where for some reason the situation always looks more dire than it does at home.

"Is there as much hair there today as last month?" you ask yourself. "That hair in the sink, in my shower drain, on my brush. Am I going bald?" As your hair starts to disappear, you feel helpless because you're at the mercy of your hair; you can't control its fallout any more than you can control the weather. To a young man of twenty-one a receding hairline can seem like the end of the world.

Is it really hopeless? Of course not! If you're just starting to lose your hair, there are many things you can do to slow its loss; if you're bald already, there are still options to replace your hair or cover up your bald pate. This book will help you, no matter what stage your hair loss is in.

Hair 101: What exactly is hair?

Most people have no idea what really lurks beneath their hair, unless they've been shaving it off already.

For something that you play with, obsess over, color, cut, and twist into odd shapes, hair is surprisingly dead. Yes, the hair you think looks so vibrant and alive is actually not alive at all. I'm not saying that you should ignore or mistreat your hair. For something that's dead, hair is quite capable of responding to good treatment or bad.

Hair is technically part of your skin, although like fingernails and toenails, it grows and separates from your skin. The average head contains around 100,000 hair follicles, and your entire body is home to around 5 million hair follicles. Most of the complex activity that keeps your hair growing goes on below the surface.

The active growth phase of a hair follicle, called the *anagen* phase, averages around three years. At any given time, about 90 percent of your hair is in the anagen phase, and the other 10 percent is taking a rest in the *telogen* phase, which is the resting phase, and disappears from your head.

Hair grows about ½ inch a month (although it certainly seems like more when you need a haircut!) and grows to a length of 1½ to 3 feet before growth stops and the hair falls out. (In Chapter 2, we tell you all you ever wanted to know about hair, right down to its roots.)

Hair 102: Why do we have hair?

Hair is more than just a pretty cover up. It serves many biological functions and actually covers most of your body (often growing in places you'd rather it didn't).

The functions of hair (both on your head and elsewhere on your body) are that

- It protects your head.
- It keeps you warm in the winter and cool in the summer.
- It protects you against sunburn.
- It has nerve endings that serve to make a scalp massage feel good, yet tell you when a mosquito has landed on your arm to bite you.

Hair and ethnicity: How race impacts hair

What your hair looks like is directly related to the genes you received from your parents. There are some hair generalities related to different racial groups, although your individual hair traits will vary. Many people's gene pool today is pretty diverse! (See Chapter 2 for much more about hair and ethnicity.)

However, the following generalities apply:

- Although it appears that many Caucasians have thinner hair than other ethnicities, Caucasians actually have the highest number of hairs on their heads, an average of two hundred hairs per square centimeter.
- Asians have the thickest and coarsest hair, which makes it appear as though they have more hairs on their head. They average a hundred and fifty hairs per square centimeter.
- African Americans have the thinnest and the finest hair, but because it mats together more than Caucasian or Asian hair, it appears thicker. African hair averages a hundred and thirty hairs per square centimeter.

You're Not Alone: Dealing with Causes of Hair Loss and the Personal Impact

When you're going bald, you may feel like you're the only one. It seems like every commercial on television features hair wafting gently in the breeze as tanned youngsters run across the beach;

you may not have the tan or the body, but those are at least theoretically obtainable, whereas lost hair seems to be just that — lost youth forever.

You're not alone, though; hair loss affects over 50 million people in the United States alone, and lest you think only men have hair loss issues, over 20 million of sufferers are women. So it's a safe bet that thousands of people are thinking the same thing you are: "I can't believe I'm going bald."

The many possible causes of hair loss

Everyone loses around 100 hairs from their head every day, but serious hair loss isn't a "one cause fits all" type of problem; many factors contribute to hair loss, and we give you the full rundown in Chapters 4 and 5. The most common causes of hair loss are listed here.

- ✔ **Genetics:** Yes, you knew it all along: It's Mom's (or Dad's) fault that you have no hair. The overwhelming majority (up to 98 percent) of men with balding fall into the genetic category. Female genetic balding occurs much less frequently, but up to 50 percent of women have hair loss related to their inherited genes. (See Chapter 4 for more on genetics and hair loss.)

  The good news is that only seven percent of men develop the most advanced balding pattern (left with just a 3 inch wreath of hair around the side and back of the head). If you've inherited this pattern, it's usually evident by the time you're 30.

  Genetic hair loss in men generally falls into one of several distinct hair loss patterns identified under the Norwood classification system (see Chapter 4). In balding men, the hair around the sides of the head almost always retains a normal, thick appearance. In women, genetic hair loss is different; for one thing, it tends to occur as overall hair thinning (including the sides of the head) rather than loss of hair on certain areas of the head.

- ✔ **Diseases:** A number of diseases as well as hormonal influences, including thyroid disease and anemia, cause hair loss. Autoimmune disease also can cause patchy hair loss. We cover these causes in Chapter 5.

- ✔ **Mechanical causes:** Mechanical hair loss is caused by external forces such as tight braiding, rubber banding, turbans, or other hair torture devices that put stress and strain on your hair.

✔ **Stress:** In some cases, stress can contribute to hair loss in those who are genetically predisposed to it or can result in a sudden loss of hair in a condition called *telogen effluvium* (read all about it in Chapter 5).

✔ **Medications:** Many medicines, most notably anabolic steroids, birth control pills, antidepressants, and tranquilizers, can cause hair loss. (See Chapter 5 for a complete list).

Society's emphasis on hair

"So what if you're going bald — it's only hair!" Statements like that can make your blood boil when you first start losing your hair. Most people are cavalier about hair loss when they're not the ones losing it and are unsympathetic to the plight of the victims of hair loss, but when their hair starts falling out, they'll be looking for miracle cures, too — you can be sure of it.

Hair loss isn't life threatening, but it can be an extreme threat to self-esteem. Studies show that hair loss can lead to feelings of shame, depression, frustration, helplessness, and anger. It also can result in feelings of sexual inadequacy and loss of self confidence.

Today, hair is something of a status symbol; you can find thousands of products devoted to hair care, which only emphasize the problem for those experiencing hair loss. Many men now have their hair styled rather than just getting it cut at a local barber shop. Television gives the impression that a full head of luxurious hair is the norm, implying that those who are losing it are somehow abnormal.

Hair is also used as a method of self expression, a way to say who you are. A "bad hair day" can ruin your week; a "no hair life" can derail your career, your love life, and your self-esteem, but so can anything, *if you let it.*

Before you can fix a problem, you have to realize you have a problem. Denial is your enemy; you can't fix what you can't admit. This book will teach you what you need to know about keeping your hair before you lose it or getting it back if you waited too long. The good news is that there are solutions to hair loss, no matter where you are in the hair loss process.

Why men worry about losing their hair

Twenty-five percent of men will show signs of balding by age 30 and 50 percent by the time they're 50. While women can rearrange their hair to help disguise hair loss or resort to extensions or wigs, men sometimes don't have enough hair — or wear it long enough — to utilize these options.

Studies have shown that self confidence levels both inside and outside of the workplace can be affected by hair loss, and that correcting hair loss can have huge psychological and career benefits.

The devastation of hair loss in women

Women lose hair, but not in the same ways as men do. However, severe hair loss can be even more devastating to women than it is to men. Hair loss may be a serious blow to a woman's self-esteem, in large part because of cultural norms, society's concept of femininity, and the expectation that a woman should have glossy, luxurious, well-kept hair. We know that because the magazines women read tell them just that.

As much as half of the female population suffers from hair loss at some time in their lives. Women's hair loss tends to differ from men's hair loss both in cause and in the way the hair is affected. Women's hair loss is generally widespread, with thinning all over the scalp rather than loss in certain areas; rarely do you see women whose hair loss leaves them bald on top with a healthy fringe around the edges like the typical look of male pattern baldness. In Chapter 4, we look at the unique challenges of hair loss in women.

For women, thinning hair may be caused by a number of medical conditions which, when treated, may restore their hair. This book covers these issues in Chapter 6.

Keeping Your Hair Healthy

In the process of caring for our hair, we do many damaging things to it, from combing it the wrong way to coloring it with harsh chemicals or subjecting it to strong sunlight.

If you're starting to lose your hair, it's important to take the best possible care of the hair you still have. Throughout this book, we discuss the best ways to care for your hair, but here a few of the worst things you can do to your hair. (See Chapter 3 for a full discussion of proper hair care).

✔ Never back comb your hair: It damages the hair shaft.

✔ Don't rub your hair dry with a towel.

✔ Don't over dry your hair with a blow dryer; stop before your hair is completely dry.

✔ Select the right shampoo and conditioner for your hair type (Chapter 3 tells you how).

Surveying Hair Replacement Options

Whether you're a man or a woman, losing your hair doesn't mean you have to present a bald head to the world; in most cases, your options range from the simple, like plopping a department store wig on your head, to the more complicated (and expensive), like pricey hair systems or hair transplant surgery.

Minimizing or hiding hair loss

In a society used to chemical fixes and instant gratification, your first response to falling hair may be to search the drugstore shelves for a tonic that will replace lost hair — or at least preserve what you still have. You want to believe that these tonics will do the job and restore your head to its former glory. There are medications that can help save your hair, but you may not want to resort to medication, at least not just yet.

Chapter 3 gives you a wealth of information on taking care of your hair because, although good hair care by itself can't help you fight genetic hair loss, it will keep your hair looking good while you still have it. In cases where hair loss results from disease or mechanical damage, good hair care can help you keep your hair as well as keep it looking good.

In Chapter 8, we introduce some of the products that can work with the hair you have left to give the illusion of fuller hair. It's not quite as simple as spraying silly string on the top of your head or using a can of paint to color your bald spot, but today's spray-on or powdery products can definitely improve your hair's appearance for some time without looking weird.

Wearing a wig

When we say "wig," we don't mean the powdered version commonly worn in the 1700s — although if that's your style, who's to stop you? In this book, we use the terms "wig" or "hair replacement system" (hair systems for short) when we are referring to a hairpiece as a hair replacement option for men or women (usually wigs for women and toupees for men, but the terminology is flexible).

Wigs have improved tremendously over the last few decades, and a good one is virtually undetectable. (Your hair stylist will know, but he or she may be the only one.)

A wig can be a quick fix for temporary hair loss, such as the hair loss from chemotherapy treatments, or it can be your lifetime solution to lost hair. Many women have several wigs and can change from "Gee, you need a haircut" to a freshly trimmed look overnight. Men may have many hair systems to wear in various settings or situations.

You can buy an inexpensive wig for less than $100, but if you want it to be foolproof, you probably have to spend more than that. A good wig (or wigs) can easily run into the thousands, and it's possible for the maintenance fees to rival those of your car or condo. Turn to Part III for all the details on buying and caring for hair replacement systems of all sorts.

Pharmaceutical, laser, and topical treatments

If hair loss looks like it's going to be a permanent part of your life, you may be ready to turn to prescription medications or treatments to minimize your losses. The good news is that treatments are available to help slow hair loss caused by inherited male pattern baldness. (See Chapter 9 for a rundown of prescription medications, Chapter 10 for a list of herbs that some people swear by, as well as dietary recommendations for maintaining a healthy scalp.)

For many women, hair loss may also respond to medication, or, if a specific disease process is causing the loss, by addressing the health issue.

Anyone can have healthier hair by modifying their diets, but giving you hair through medication is a bit more selective. Medications have limitations and may only work on certain types of hair loss.

They can be used in addition to surgical procedures, such as hair transplant, to help slow continuing hair loss (yes, you still lose hair after a transplant — not the transplanted hair, but hair in balding areas) or to help you keep your hair as long as possible.

Zapping your head with lasers to help your hair grow may sound like science fiction, but some laser treatments can do just that. Chapter 11 has information on which laser treatments may help and which ones will part you from your money without adding a hair to your head.

Considering hair restoration surgery

Hair transplants were an option out of reach for many men until fairly recently. With new advances in technology and better access to well-trained surgeons who work with modern techniques, the option of transplant is more accessible — and more men are taking advantage of it.

Around 100,000 American men have hair transplants every year, and the results are truly remarkable. What's most impressive is that these men look so natural that not even their hairdresser will know for sure!

The difficulties of transplants in the past — the pluggy look — have been largely overcome with better technologies and well-trained surgeons. The main objection to a hair transplant is the cost, which is why it's vitally important that you pick a hair transplant surgeon who will give you the most for your money in terms of positive, long-lasting results.

Although the cost of a hair transplant can sound exorbitant at first glance, it may not be as far out of your reach as you think. The fact is that a hair transplant costs less than five years' worth of buying and maintaining one decent quality wig!

We devote Chapter 13 to advising you on how to choose a hair transplant surgeon (price should never be your main consideration!), take you through the transplant process, and go home with you and your new hair in Chapter 14 to look at how life will be after your transplant.

Looking at the Future of Hair Loss Prevention

The future of hair loss prevention is bright. Surgical procedures are improving all the time (the transplant surgeon of tomorrow may be a robot!), and new medications are being developed to slow or at times reverse hair loss. Gene manipulation and hair cloning may not be too far down the road to give you an unlimited amount of hair to work with.

In the meantime, hair replacement systems are better looking than ever, and more research has been done on hair care products and treatments and ways to enhance the hair you have. Chapter 12 takes a look at what's on the hair horizon and the techniques that could make hair loss a thing of the past.

Chapter 2

Splitting Hairs: Growth, Loss, and Change over Time

*N*ot all hair is the same. Some people have thick, some thin; some is beautifully blonde, some is a glossy black; some is shiny, some is dull. Depending upon where hair is on your body, some grows long and some short, some is straight and some curly. Knowing more about the characteristics of hair and what type of hair you have is particularly important when your hair thins and falls out because coverage and the appearance of fullness in a balding person critically depends upon the characteristics of the hair and skin color.

Although understanding some of the factors that contribute to hair loss can't necessarily help prevent the loss, understanding the fundamental relationships between hair and skin color, hair density, bulk, and other characteristics can help you maximize the fullness you can achieve as well as guide you in your replacement options.

In this chapter, we explain the parts of a single follicle and hair shaft, how hair grows, the different hair types, what causes those differences, and some factors that can slow its growth, including age and ethnicity. We share all this with you to arm you with the knowledge you need to assess your own hair situation and investigate the options available to you to deal with it — whether you're thinking about replacement or transplantation or just creative hairstyling.

Under the Microscope: Hair and Scalp Anatomy

Hair is much more complex than it looks. In this section, we describe how hair follicles grow and alter with time and other factors. Understanding how hair follicles function (and what makes them stop functioning) can help you maintain them, thereby slowing the hair loss process.

Going beneath the skin

Most people think of hair only in terms of what they see above the scalp, but hair is actually a rather complex organ that goes beneath the surface. Anatomically speaking, hair is part of your skin. But because hair is physically distinct from skin, it's referred to as a *skin appendage*. (Other skin appendages include sweat glands, fingernails, and toenails.) See Figure 2-1.

Skin is composed of three main layers:

- **The epidermis:** This outer layer of the skin is less than 1 millimeter thick. It's composed of dead cells that are in a constant state of sloughing and replacement. As dead cells are lost, new ones from the growing layer below replace them.

- **The dermis:** This tough layer of connective tissue is about 2 to 3 millimeters thick on the scalp. This layer gives the skin its strength and contains both sebaceous (oil) glands and sweat glands.

  Sebaceous glands produce an oily substance, which creates a plug of wax (sebum) to cover the opening to the growing hair follicle. As the hair grows upward from the skin surface, some of the waxy substance is taken up by the hair shaft as a lubricant, giving the hair a waxy sheen.

  Sweat glands help control body temperature, particularly when it's hot. These glands produce a watery, salty sweat; as the sweat evaporates, body heat is lost.

- **Subcutaneous fat and connective tissue:** This layer contains the larger sensory nerve branches and the blood vessels that nourish the skin. In the scalp, the lower portions of the hair follicles (called the *bulbs*) are found in the upper part of this fatty layer.

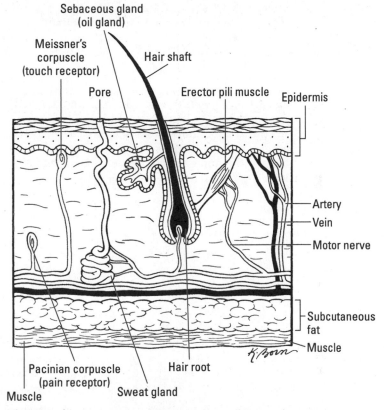

Sebaceous gland
(oil gland)

Meissner's
corpuscle
(touch receptor)

Hair shaft

Pore

Erector pili muscle

Epidermis

Artery

Vein

Motor nerve

Subcutaneous
fat

Muscle

Pacinian corpuscle
(pain receptor)

Hair root

Muscle

Sweat gland

Figure 2-1: The "hair organ" made up a hair follicle and all the structures that support it.

Dissecting a hair follicle

The hair follicle must function properly in order to maintain a healthy head of hair. A hair follicle is a complex structure that measures about 4 to 6 millimeters in length. Each follicle produces one to four hair shafts, each about 0.1 millimeters in width (in other words, these are really, really tiny structures).

The layers of a hair follicle

Hair follicles have three layers surrounding the strand of hair, which you can see in Figure 2-2:

> ✔ **The outer root sheath, or trichelemma:** This is the outer layer, which surrounds the follicle in the dermis and then blends into the epidermis on the surface of the skin, forming the pore from which the hair grows.

✔ **The inner root sheath:** This middle layer is composed of three parts, with the cuticle being the innermost portion that touches the strand of hair. The cuticle of the inner root sheath interlocks with the hair cuticle (described in "the layers of the hair shaft" section) to give it rigidity.

✔ **The bulb:** This is the lower portion of each hair follicle. It contains the inner *matrix cells,* which produce bundles (also called spindles) of hair cells that look like fine wires in an electric cord. These bundles are actually made up of even smaller bundles, which literally twist as they're made. The size of the bulb and the number of matrix cells determine the width of the fully grown hair.

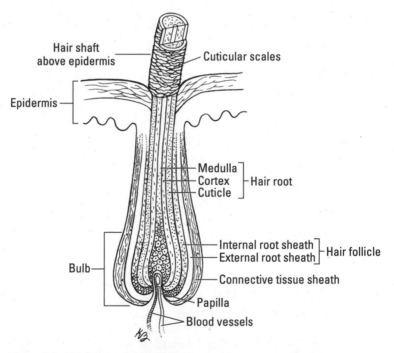

Hair shaft above epidermis

Cuticular scales

Epidermis

Medulla
Cortex — Hair root
Cuticle

Internal root sheath
External root sheath — Hair follicle

Bulb

Connective tissue sheath

Papilla

Blood vessels

Figure 2-2: The layers of the hair shaft.

The layers of the hair shaft

The hair shaft is composed of three layers.

✔ **The cuticle:** This layer forms the surface of the hair and is what you see as the hair shaft emerges from the follicle.

✔ **The cortex:** This middle layer comprises the bulk of the hair shaft and is what gives hair its strength. It's composed of an organic protein called *keratin,* the same material that comprises rhinoceros horns and deer antlers.

✔ **The medullas:** This is the center, or core, of the hair shaft, and it's only present in terminal hair follicles (a fully grown hair).

The dermal papillae

At the bottom of the hair follicle, there is a bulbous (bulb) portion which contains a small collection of specialized cells called the *dermal papillae.* Scientists believe these cells are at least partially responsible for determining. how long the hair will eventually grow, how thick it will be, and the character of the hair will be.

For many years, scientists thought that hair actually grew from the dermal papillae. Recent evidence shows that the growth center is not totally controlled from the dermal papillae. Elements that control hair growth can be found all the way up to the region of the follicle where the sebaceous glands are attached.

If the dermal papillae is removed (which sometimes happens during a hair transplant (see Chapter 13), the hair follicle may still be able to regenerate new hair, although the new hair may not be a characteristically healthy looking terminal hair. It may be shorter, thinner, and more kinky or wavy.

How hair grows

Hair doesn't grow in individual strands but rather emerges from the scalp in groups of one to four (and sometimes even five or six) strands. Hair follicles are arranged in the skin in naturally occurring groups called *follicular units*.

At any given time, about 90 percent of a person's terminal hairs are actively growing. This growth phase, called *anagen,* can last for two to seven years, though the average is about three. Scalp hair grows at an average rate of about 0.44 millimeters a day, or about ½ inch per month.

The 10 percent of scalp hairs not actively growing are in a resting state called *telogen* that, in a healthy scalp, lasts about three to five months. When a hair enters its resting phase, growth stops, the bulb detaches from the papilla, and the shaft is either pulled out (as when combing one's hair) or pushed out when the new shaft starts to grow.

Hairs grow in naturally growing groups of one to four hairs each. These are called follicular units. The follicular unit has two types of hair. The terminal hair and a vellus hair or two. These vellus hairs are smaller, shorter, and finer than the terminal hairs found in the follicular unit.

When a hair falls out on its own, a small black bulb can often be seen at the end of the hair. If it's pulled out while it is in its growth (anagen) phase, it will produce pain when it is pulled out and a white, sticky mucus swelling will often be seen at the bottom of the hair shaft. Most people assume that this is the growth center of the hair and that pulling it out means the hair won't grow again.

But cells of the dermal papillae and the growth centers found along the side of the hair shaft near the sebaceous gland will remain in the place after the hair is pulled out. These cells will multiply and cause a new hair to grow at the same location in a month or so. So pulling out a single hair should not kill that hair.

Humans lose about 100 hairs per day. The presence of a much larger number of hairs on your comb, in the sink, or in the tub can be the first sign of excessive hair loss. We become sensitized by balding in our family history and a thinning appearance on the scalp. Although we may see hair in the drain often, if we are not balding or thinning we might think nothing of it.

Letting down your hair

You're probably familiar with the Grimm's fairy tale about Rapunzel, a young maid who was put into a high tower when she was a girl. One day, a prince heard her crying and was smitten by her beauty and her long blonde braided hair. When he couldn't find a door into the tower to rescue her, he asked that she let down her golden hair so he could climb up and rescue her. The beautiful Rapunzel let her hair hang over the edge of the tower, and the prince scurried up to her rescue. After some harrowing events, they lived happily ever after.

It's a good story but, notwithstanding freakish exceptions (the current world record hair length is more than 18 feet), clearly the Brothers Grimm weren't well-versed in the biology of normal hair growth. They couldn't have known that the longest growth phase of hair is growth was six or seven years, making Rapunzel's hair a maximum of about 1 meter in length (that's six or seven years at ½ inch per month). Certainly, Rapunzel could have jumped from a height of 1 meter, but if she had, the Brothers Grimm wouldn't have had much of a story for the millions of children who wanted to believe in the magic of the prince who rescues the fair maid. Ignorance is bliss!

Linking Ethnicity with Hair Type and Loss

People aren't all created equally — with respect to hair. Ethnicity and race affect your hair type and density, as we explain for the three ethnic groups in the following list. Keep in mind that although certain ethnicities are more likely to have a certain type and density of hair, variations do exist. There simply isn't enough space in this book for us to go into that much detail.

Why should you know about the connection between your ethnicity and the type of hair on your head? Hair is a specialized organ system probably related, in some cases, to the climates we're born into. For example, the African's dark skin protects against strong sunlight and sun burns, and his kinky hair becomes an efficient heat exchanger to keep the body cool while providing some shade from the hot sun.

There are, however, no explanations for the typically straight, lower density hair of Asians when compared to Caucasians, or the high density hair counts of many Northern Europeans.

✔ **Caucasian hair:** Generally, Caucasians have the highest number of hairs on their scalp. The density of hair on a typical Caucasian averages 200 hairs per one square centimeter.

A healthy Caucasian human scalp contains about 100,000 follicles that produce thicker terminal hairs. (In comparison, the human body has approximately five million non-scalp follicles that produce the fine, *vellus* hair scattered around the body.)

Caucasian hair generally appears thick because it's more difficult to see through to the scalp than on Asians and Africans.

✔ **Asian hair:** Asians have fewer scalp hairs than Caucasians, with about 140 to 160 hairs per square centimeter on the average. A healthy Asian human scalp contains about 80,000 follicles.

Asian hair tends to be straight and with a low density. Visually, it doesn't cover the head as well as the curly or wavy hair of Caucasians. But some Asians have the coarsest and thickest hairs, which can offset their lower hair density.

Visually, straight Asian hair just doesn't cover well, and with their lower densities, the problem of see through hair is compounded.

✔ **African/African American hair:** Of the three groups we outline here, African Americans have the lowest density of hair, ranging from 120 to 140 hairs per square centimeter. A healthy African or African American human scalp contains about 60,000 follicles.

Some Africans and African Americans actually have fine hairs, and some is kinkier than others. Because African hair often sticks together, it may appear that there's more hair despite the low hair densities that are characteristic of all Africans and African Americans. Africans generally have a dark skin which obscures the lower densities because of the low contrast between hair and skin color.

Aging Hair: How It Changes with Time

Like the rest of you, your hair is impacted by age, sometimes for the better, and other times, for the worse. There's nothing you can do to stop time from marching on in your hair cells, but knowing what changes to expect can help you plan for ways to compensate for them through the use of hair growth stimulating medications, by styling changes.

Knowing what's normal and what's not as you age may also help you recognize early genetic hair loss and plan to treat it early, as medications and transplantation work best when you still have enough hair to work with.

Change of texture

Whether a baby's hair sticks up all over or forms only a few wispy curls, all baby hair is baby fine. But hair changes during childhood. It remains soft but becomes bulkier. Through the teenage years and into early adulthood, hair takes on an adult texture, becoming coarser as a rule.

Hair counts are thought to be maintained well into the senior years, at least for half of the human population. The other half experiences hair loss prior to reaching their 50s.

The weight of each individual hair shaft is genetically imprinted in your genes, as is the number of hairs you're born with. It's not unusual for an adult to start off with a medium-coarse hair shaft, only to find that as he or she ages, the hair becomes finer as the thickness of the hair shaft changes in adulthood.

This change is slow and, provided that the number of hairs on the head doesn't drop off precipitously, the change usually isn't alarming.

Of those men who have a full head of hair into their 60s, nearly half will experience a substantial reduction in the thickness of each individual hair shaft.

One in three women will also experience an overall pattern of thinning hair in menopause, due to an increased sensitivity to the male hormone testosterone.

Loss of hair

The presence of baldness genes and the hormone DHT (see Chapter 4 for more on DHT and its role in hair loss) alone aren't enough to cause baldness. Even after a person has reached maturity, susceptible hair follicles must continually be exposed to the hormone over a period of time for hair loss to occur. The age at which these effects finally manifest themselves varies from one individual to another and is related to a person's genetic composition and to the levels of testosterone in the bloodstream.

Although balding can start in men in their teens, it's unusual to see it much before the age of 17, when there appears to be a genetic switch that starts the process. For example, a 15 year old may have a full head of hair until, all of a sudden, he passes an age in the later teens (usually between 17 and 19) and a genetic switch is flipped on and he starts losing his hair.

Hair loss doesn't occur all at once, nor does it occur in a steady, straight-line progression. People losing their hair experience alternating periods of slow and rapid hair loss and even note periods of stability. Many of the factors that cause the rate of loss to speed up or slow down are unknown, but it's proven that with age, a person's total hair volume decreases.

Even if there's no predisposition to genetic balding, some hairs randomly begin to shrink in width and not grow as long as a person ages. As a result, each group of hairs contains both full terminal hairs and thinner hairs (similar to the finer hairs that grow on the rest of the body), making the scalp look less full.

Eventually, some of the thinner hairs are lost, and the actual number of follicular units may be reduced (for an explanation of follicular units, refer to the earlier section, "How hair grows"). In about one third of adults, even the hair around the back and side of the head (the fringe area) gradually thins over time.

Fortunately, in most people, the fringe areas of hair retain enough permanent hair to make hair transplantation possible — even for a patient well into his 70s or 80s! In a small number of men, however, the process of hair aging may start in the 20s or 30s, resulting in a uniformly falling hair count. When this happens, transplantation is more difficult because there's not enough donor hair left to cover balding areas.

Hair through thick and thin

Some heads of hair appear thicker than others. The thickness of the hair shaft is a factor in how full hair appears: A coarse, thicker hair shaft has more bulk than a finer hair shaft. The texture is also very important.

In Caucasians, heavy, coarse hair isn't a common trait, but if you have it, your hair appears very, very thick. People with fine, thin hair often have a "see-through" look, particularly in bright light, even if they're not balding; a natural higher density may offset this look to some degree.

A good way to tell whether hair shafts have lost bulk between childhood and adulthood is to think back to your childhood memories. We always ask patients the following question: "When you were about 10 years old, do you remember members of your family rubbing your hair for good luck?" With the 10 year old with coarse hair, every aunt and uncle coming for a visit would rub his hair for good luck, commenting on his healthy head of hair. People who don't recall this generally didn't have coarse hair.

So when we see a man with see-through hair but normal hair densities, this question can illuminate the changes in hair bulk as aging occurs.

We've seen fair-skinned individuals color their hair to a lighter color so that the contrast between their hair and skin color is minimized, making their hair look distinctly fuller. When hair and skin have similar colors (such as blonde hair on white skin), the coverage appears fuller than if there's a high contrast in the colors (such as black hair against white skin).

In a hair transplant, this contrast may dictate the surgical techniques employed by the surgeon and the amount of hair that needs to be moved in order to obtain a fuller look.

Chapter 3

Taking Better Care of Your Hair

*H*air can be your crowning glory. Through the ages, people have primped, crimped, colored, and pampered their locks. Hair care products promising the wildest results overflow store shelves. According to some commercials, the right shampoo can change your life.

Even though you know that vibrant hair isn't really going to change your life all that much, it can make you feel better about yourself, increase your confidence, and maybe even get you a few compliments. Treating your hair well helps avoid damage that can result in permanent hair loss, and it helps you keep the hair you have for as long as possible.

In this chapter, we look at some structural qualities of your hair as well as hair care products commonly used today. You find out how the different ways styling and enhancing your hair can damage it, and along the way, we explain how to go about kinder, gentler hair care.

Although this chapter describes general hair care tips, the purpose of including it in *Hair Loss & Replacement For Dummies* is to let you know how proper hair care and various products can help slow the hair loss process, help maintain the best quality of the hair you have, and disguise your thinning hair.

Admiring the Adaptable Qualities of Hair

This may come as a surprise to you, but the hair on your head is dead. Don't feel too bad, though — everyone else's hair is dead, too. So why waste time taking care of something that's dead? And if it's not alive, then how can you make your hair look better — or last longer?

Even though your hair is dead, how you treat it *can* make it look much better — or worse — because hair has many attributes of a living organ and can repair itself under the right conditions.

Stripping away the coating: Inside your hair

It's easier to care for your hair properly if you understand how the individual parts of a human hair are affected by the way you care for it. In this section, we look at the anatomy of a human hair.

Cutting into a hair

Hair is made up of dead compressed cells produced about ¼ inch below the skin. At the end of each hair is the hair bulb, which is essentially the factory for making the hair; this part of the hair is alive and working all the time. Each hair has its own bulb, and damage to the hair bulb can result in permanent loss of that hair. (Turn to Chapter 2 for a look at the anatomy of a hair follicle.)

Each individual hair can be compared to an electrical wire. If you cut into a wire, you see that it has a rubbery outer covering and twisted or bundled inner wires that carry electricity. Human hair is made up of an outer covering called the *cuticle* that contains individual bundles of hair called the *cortex*. The cuticle gives the hair shaft a round or oval shape. Stripping off the cuticle would leave the hair looking like a series of out of control wires.

The bundles (also called *spindles*) of hair cells in the cortex are actually made up of even smaller bundles that literally twist as they're made. With African American hair, the hair cells are so heavily twisted (up to 12 times more twists per length than Caucasian hair) as the bundles are made that the hair is kinky. The tight twists tend to kink the cuticle, producing pointed, vulnerable edges that make the hair more susceptible to damage. The less the twists, the straighter the hair.

Combing the cuticles

The outer layer of the hair, the cuticle, protects the inner spindles and bundles. The cuticle has scales that, like scales on a fish or shingles on your roof, protect the hair within. When you take a knife against the grain of scales on a fish, you take off the scales; with the hair cuticle, imagine your fingers or comb rubbing against the direction of the cuticle scales doing the same type of damage.

The scales make the cuticle porous, allowing the hair to breathe. This is very important because the ability to hydrate hair depends upon the porous nature of the cuticle. The scales also relate to how the hair feels: When you stroke it one way, it feels smooth, and the other way there's a roughness to it.

Breaking the hair bonds

The bonds that help hold hair in a certain position can be broken or rearranged, such as when hair is permed or straightened. There are three types of bonds that determine the strength and the lift of the hair:

- ✔ **Hydrogen bonds:** These bonds break down easily and give hair its flexibility. Hydrogen bonds come apart when you wet your hair and come back together again as your hair dries.

- ✔ **Salt bonds:** These are temporary and easy to rearrange because they're water-dependent and easily dissolved when your hair is washed. Salt bonds are easily broken by weak alkaline products like ammonia or acid solutions that contain chlorine or copper peptide in high concentration and by changes in pH. These bonds can be reformed by normalizing the pH level of the hair with normalizing solutions available at your local hair salons.

- ✔ **Disulfide bonds:** These are relatively permanent and can only be changed with perming and relaxing agents. Disulphide bonds are stronger than hydrogen and salt bonds, and there are fewer of them than the other types. Disulfide bonds are the most important factors in supplying the hair with its strength and durability, and as such, they can't be broken by heat or water.

Wet hair can be stretched by as much as 30 percent, and you can change the shape of the hair bonds when it's stretched. For example, when you put rollers on your wet hair and then allow the hair to dry on the rollers, the hydrogen bonds take on the shape of the rollers, which essentially sets the hydrogen bonds in this new shape.

Keeping it greased: Sebum's role in healthy hair

Your scalp helps keep your hair looking healthy by supplying an abundant and constant production of *sebum,* a waxy material made by sebaceous glands. It's secreted onto the hair as it emerges from the scalp through pores in the skin. The sebum works its way into the hair on the surface of the cuticle, and it's spread through the hair as the hair moves in the wind, by combing it, touching it, and by hairs rubbing against other adjacent hairs.

If hair is cut short, the same amount of sebum is produced, so relatively more sebum covers less hair, causing it to appear more greasy. (It also causes the bald pate to acquire a sheen rather quickly after showering because there's no hair to carry off the oil.) There's nothing you can do about oily hair other than wash your hair more often and use a shampoo made especially for greasy hair.

 Adolescents have unusually high sebum output, which is why so many teenagers complain of greasy or oily hair. We're often asked to prescribe drugs to decrease sebum production in teenagers who hate their greasy hair. Some professionals feel that the sebum production can be impacted by drugs such as Propecia or saw palmetto (an herb; see Chapter 10), which block production of the DHT hormone, but studies show no connection between a lack of DHT production and decreased sebum production.

Choosing and Using the Right Products

The right shampoo and conditioner can work wonders on your hair, helping it stay not only shiny and attractive but also healthy. With shelves and shelves of products available in stores, how do you know which ones to choose? Should you go for the one with the most four-syllable ingredients on the label, or maybe the one with the label that coordinates with your bathroom colors? Or are they all the same, and the cheapest will do?

In this section, we help you pick out products that will benefit your hair, as well as describe the improvements that science has brought to the world of hair care products and how they affect you and your locks.

Remembering the "no wash" years

For centuries, hair care was a time consuming, uncomfortable process that often did more harm than good. Before shampoo was invented, harsh soaps, often made of animal fats, were used to scrub the hair in much the same way as you scrub your hands today to clean them. The washing process left scummy soap deposits sticking to the hair, which made it look dull. Scrubbing got the dirt out, but with varying degrees of damage in the process.

Because hair washing in the old days was a major ordeal for many people, particularly women with long hair, it wasn't unusual to avoid the process until such a time as it became impossible to ignore. The unwashed hair built up sebum (grease), which stuck to the 100 to 150 hairs shed daily and flakes of shed skin. This all resulted in the hair becoming matted overnight. Tossing and turning in one's sleep resulted in a semi-permanent "bed head" as mats of hair became cemented to each other.

The result not only looked bad, but it also smelled pretty ghastly. People tried to manage the problem with powders to hide the visuals and perfumes to mask the odors. These powders added more particulate matter to the mats of hair and sebum, making the problem much worse in the long run. So if you've ever lamented the fact that you need to wash your hair regularly, be thankful that you can do just that!

Looking at today's hair care products

Things have definitely changed for the better in the industrialized world. Today, it's not unusual to wash your hair frequently, sometimes more than once a day. Although this is a good move from both a visual and an odor perspective, it means that modern shampoos must be designed to prevent damage incurred by frequent use.

Shampooing your hair removes environmental particles that may build up during your daily activities. People who work in dirty environments (such as shoveling coal in a coal mine) or even just outside all day will clearly build up more particulate matter than those people who work indoors. Cleaning your hair removes any particulate matter as well as the sebum that builds up throughout the day.

Attracting positive products to your hair

You probably never knew this, but hair has a small negative electric charge. Thinking back to high school chemistry, you may remember that opposite charges attract. That means that you can use chemicals and products that have a positive charge to them in an effort to treat mild damage to your hair. These products are attracted to the negatively charged hair and coat the hair cuticle, restoring the shine to dull, dry hair and making it more manageable.

One product that can help your hair through electricity is conditioner, which carries a weak positive charge. The positive molecules in the conditioner, which contains silicone, stick to the negatively charged hair shafts, and the conditioner molecules penetrate the scales of the cuticle, allowing moisture to reach the matrix of the hair shaft. This moisture increases the hair's shine and luster and the depth of the hair color.

Add this to the conditioning properties that help detangle the hair when combing it, and you get conditioners that make hair softer and easier to manage — wet or dry.

Getting the tangles out

Most modern shampoos also contain some conditioning agents mixed in with the cleansers for easy combing of wet hair. You also have the option of using a separate conditioner for even better detangling.

If you're having difficulty detangling your hair, applying more and more conditioner won't help. Rather, dry your hair and then use a detangling agent.

Dreadlocks or long kinky hair can be a detangling nightmare. It may help to separate your hair into sections and go through each section using a long knitting needle. Detangle it from the scalp outward if possible; you may run into a knot that you need to detangle against the direction of the scales on the cuticle.

Damage to the hair structure during the detangling process is a real risk, so this process should never be rushed. In other words, attempting to yank your comb through a tangle is a hair care no-no.

Adding chemicals

Shampoos and conditioners are more than cleaning agents: They're also an alphabet soup of chemicals. Various chemicals are added to

- Control the viscosity (thickness of the solution).
- Control the pH (the degree of acidity present).

✔ Act as preservation agents to ensure that bacteria doesn't grow in the shampoos and conditioners.

✔ Make the products attractive. Coloring agents are used in conjunction with perfumes to make the product please both your eyes and your nose.

Hair care products often include chemicals such as dimethicone and panthenol (a vitamin B derivative), which are absorbed into the hair shaft and provide moisture to dry areas when the new hair grows. These compounds are more easily absorbed by the hair when surfactants are also added to the mix (see the section "Keeping things slippery with surfactants" in this chapter for more); surfactants help overcome the body's sebum, which can prevent full absorption of moisture in the hair.

Certain shampoos contain compounds like zinc pyrithione to treat flaky scalps (otherwise known as *dandruff*). These shampoos generally state on the packaging whether they're recommended for people with dandruff. All shampoos that claim to treat dandruff must meet FDA over-the-counter drug requirements.

Volumizing shampoos and conditioners that add moisture to the hair shaft, thereby increasing the bulk of the hair, contain such unpronounceable products as polyquarternium and stearamidaproply dimethylamine, which alter the electric charge on the hair shaft. These tongue twisters are particularly important in winter months when the air is dry, especially in heated buildings.

Keeping things slippery with surfactants

Today's commercial shampoos contain compounds called *surfactants*, compounds that accomplish a number of things when added to shampoo. Surfactants

✔ Help shampoo lather up in hard or soft water.

✔ Help hair rinse easily and thoroughly.

✔ Eliminate the need for hard scrubbing, which can damage your hair.

✔ Facilitate removal of grease and any dirt from the scalp and hair, because the surfactant can penetrate physical barriers, such as flakes of skin and dirt, embedded in the skin or hair.

✔ Facilitate the foaming properties of a shampoo, which helps lift the particulate materials (dirt) into the foam. A thicker shampoo with surfactants in it will easily spread through the hair.

✔ Maintain a balance between the penetrating power of the shampoo and the sensitivity of the scalp skin, which benefits people with sensitive skin.

Picking the proper shampoo

You have a myriad of shampoo options, but selecting the right one for your hair isn't really that difficult when you understand the categories. Shampoos are generally geared toward use on normal, fine, or dry hair; you just have to figure out which one you have. Here's a breakdown:

✔ **Normal hair**

- Is neither greasy nor dry.
- Isn't permed or color treated.
- Generally holds its style well, without the use of lots of products.
- Looks good most of the time.

✔ **Fine hair**

- Tends to be limp.
- Looks flat and lacks volume.
- Is difficult to manage.
- Becomes greasy soon after it's washed.

✔ **Dry hair**

- Is dull.
- Is frizzy.
- Feels rough.
- Has been treated with perms or coloring agents.
- Tangles easily.

Excess oils tend to weigh the hair down, making it difficult to manage, because the oil clings to dirt and particulate matter. Because sebum is easily spread by passing your fingers through your hair, don't run your fingers through your hair after you finish drying and styling it.

And if your hair is greasy, be sure to use a shampoo designed for greasy hair. It has more powerful surfactants to get the grease off of the scalp and hair shafts, but be aware that more powerful surfactants may be more irritating to the eyes and skin.

Knowing when to trust the label

Because the FDA is involved in the regulation of claims on the labels and the advertising material on these products, you can generally trust the claims if the company is well known. On the other hand, many fly-by-night companies will risk making incredible claims, hoping to fly under the FDA radar, to get you to buy their product. These products often show up on late night infomercials and feature someone wearing a white lab coat (who almost assuredly is not a doctor, although you're meant to think he is).

Because hair products don't have to be cleared by the FDA before they go on the market, there's no central place to go to find out if a product is safe and their ads are truthful. If the FDA finds that the product is being falsely advertised, they will first act by serving the company a "cease and desist" letter. It can take considerable time before a company removes a product from the market under these circumstances.

The safety and effectiveness of these products may not have been rigorously tested and you don't want to become a victim of some possibly unsafe product while waiting for the FDA to answer a complaint and then put them out of business; the best thing to do is to buy products from companies that are well known rather than those that advertise on late night TV.

Shampoos don't alter the physical properties of the hair, so hair will be just as pliable and strong after a shampoo as it was before. But conditioners in the shampoo can interfere with perming and coloring. You can offset the impact by using shampoos that contain silicone micro-emulsifiers.

Washing and drying your hair correctly

You may not think you need instructions for washing your hair, but there's a right way and a wrong way to do everything, including washing and drying your hair! Follow these instructions and you'll end up with less hair damage and healthier, better-looking hair:

1. **Wet your hair with plain warm water.**

2. **Put the shampoo in your hands and rub them together to get the lather up before applying it to your hair.**

3. **Work the shampoo into the scalp and massage gently with your finger tips to get the lather up.**

4. **Let your hair hang while you rinse it thoroughly.**

   If you're in a bath tub, lean your head forward as you rinse the shampoo out with warm water.

5. **If you're not using a shampoo that contains conditioner, put a separate conditioner in your hands and apply it to the scalp first before working it into the hair. Leave it on for at least a couple of minutes and then rinse thoroughly with warm water.**

   Shampoos combined with conditioners can be very effective for most men with short hair and for hair that's not damaged.

6. **Towel-dry your hair gently by patting it; don't rub your scalp and hair briskly with the towel and don't blow-dry your hair when soaking wet.**

7. **Comb or brush your wet hair gently. If you use a conditioner properly, the tangles should be relatively easy to take out with a wide-toothed plastic comb or brush.**

8. **If you use a mousse, gel, or setting agent, it's best applied after you pat-dry your hair, when the hair is still damp.**

   So-called *wet gels* give the hair a glossy appearance.

9. **If you blow-dry your hair, don't do so when the hair is soaking wet.**

   If you use a blow-dryer, be sure to keep it moving constantly so that the heat isn't concentrated in one area of your hair. It's always best to use the lowest heat and the lowest speed you can get away with because high heat causes hair damage. Also, damage generally occurs at the end of the blow-drying cycle, so always turn off the drier before your hair is completely dry.

How Gels, Sprays, and Other Chemicals Impact Hair Shape

Hair sprays, gels, perms, and other chemical products and processes exist for only one reason: So you can force your hair to do what you want. It's part of human nature to want what you don't have. People with straight hair want curls and people with curly hair are constantly trying to tame it into straight submission. Hair, however, has a mind of its own and has certain built-in characteristics that must be overcome if you want it to do your bidding. Some factors that influence the look of your hair are:

✔ The thickness of the hair shafts

✔ The density of the hair

✔ The natural stiffness of the hair (which keeps it from lying on the scalp like a wet noodle)

✔ The natural curvature of the hair

✔ The slippery nature of the hair (how it slides over its neighboring hairs)

✔ The cohesiveness of the hair (how it sticks to other hairs)

This section looks at the ways changing your look with chemical products and processes can also change the composition of your hair — for better, for worse, and sometimes forever.

Thickening your hair

Who wants flat, wimpy hair, the kind that lacks body or bounce? Limp hair is almost always very fine hair, because fine hair shafts don't have enough thickness to maintain their stiffness and to stand away from the scalp. Hair that's naturally curved takes up more room and makes hair appear fuller than it actually is. (People from Mediterranean areas, such as France, Spain, and Italy, are famous for lush, wavy, full-bodied hair.)

Using styling gels or a mousse that attach to your hair shafts can give your hair a thicker appearance, even if "flat as a pancake" describes your normal hair to a T. Gels and mousses increase the roughness of the hair in addition to giving the appearance of a thicker hair shaft.

The increased roughness of the hairs makes them bond to each other, which makes your hair appear fuller. When your hair is fine, it's not a good idea to use smoothing products that take away the rough character of the hair because your hair can end up appearing even thinner than it actually is.

 You may have to try several different mousses and gels to find what works best for your hair because there are so many products on the market that you need to experiment to find the one that fits you needs best). Mousses and some gels are particularly good for fine hair to increase the sense of hair bulk.

Reshaping hair

Setting can help you reshape your hair's natural appearance by giving it more volume. Blow-drying with a round brush to form the hair and then using rollers to hold it in position until the drying is complete is a common setting technique.

Setting wet hair with the help of a foam or gel increases the curvature of the hair shaft. Shampooing helps this process because surfactants in the shampoo penetrate the hair shaft, making the dried hair respond better to what you're doing to it. (Refer to the earlier section, "Keeping things slippery with surfactants," for more on these compounds in shampoo.)

Teasing hair is a common method of increasing volume, but repeated teasing will permanently damage the hair because it breaks the scales off the hair cuticle, and these broken scales can't repair themselves. (The section, "Combing the cuticles," earlier in this chapter explains the cuticles and scales.)

All the following materials are useful in setting hair because they create adhesion of the hairs. They form films on the hair shafts that dry and hold one hair to another (like a weld on the hair), producing a better lift and therefore a better illusion of volume and fullness.

✔ **Water-based materials such as gels, mousses, and foams:** These wash off easily with a good shampoo.

✔ **Hair spray:** Hair spray forms a hard film that bonds the hair into place. Combing sprayed hair that has dried can break the hair at the bonding point. Therefore, it's best not to mess with the hair after you apply hair spray, or if you do attempt to restyle it, be very careful not to tug on the hair as you comb it again.

Many people spray on way more hair spray than needed, leaving the hair overly saturated and making it very difficult to remove the hair spray completely with one shampoo application.

✔ **Hair waxes and pomades:** These are more complex to apply and much more difficult to remove, but a good strong shampoo with a very active surfactant will clean waxes and pomades off the hair shafts, although it may take more than one washing.

The advantage of waxes and pomades is that they stay in place and hold the hair against wind and even rain because they're not water-soluble. Waxes act like a plaster cast, imparting a rigidity to the hair shaft, and they work well in hair of any length. The spiked hair of many movie and rock stars is achieved using waxes and pomades.

Unlike hair-sprayed hair, which is difficult to remold, wax-based products make it easy to rework the shape of the hair again and again. They're so durable that you could restyle your hair as you walked down the street (although you may prefer to do it in front of a mirror)!

Changing Your Natural Look: Dyeing and Processing

More than half of people over age 50 have gray hair, but you'd never know it. More people dye their hair to look younger than do any other age-defying beauty enhancement. But if you want to keep your hair as long as possible, it pays to be careful with dyes, because improper use of dyes can do permanent damage to your hair.

Graying generally starts at the temples and then spreads to other parts of the scalp. Contrary to urban legend, your hair can't turn white overnight, although it may seem like it does when you let too much time elapse between coloring!

Dyeing your hair can take years off you — but it can also be bad for your hair. Plant-based dyes such as henna are less likely to cause irritation, but the color doesn't last as long as if you use chemical dyes.

Most commercial hair dyes today contain the chemical para-Phenylenediamine (PPD) as an active ingredient. It's not uncommon to develop skin sensitivity to permanent dyes containing PPD, so be sure to test the product on a small area before covering your whole head with hair color for the first time. Always check for the presence of PPD in the dye that you are going to use. Even though semi permanent dyes are not supposed to have PPD in them, never assume this for your own safety.

There are two types of patch testing for PPD:

✔ Apply a 20-percent dilution of the dye being tested to a small area on your neck below the collar; wait a full 72 hours to see if there's a reaction, which would mean a sensitivity to PPD. A reaction produces a reddened, rashy, or inflamed area of skin in the area covered by the test solution.

✔ Apply a patch containing a 2 percent concentration of PPD in a petrolatum base to the skin and leave it there for up to three days. If a rash or reddening occurs, remove the patch.

Sensitivities may arise even if you've been using a dye containing PPD for years, so not being sensitive initially to the PPD doesn't mean that you won't become sensitive to it over time.

How nature colors hair

Two types of pigment (called *melanin*) in the hair bulb create hair color, which is produced below the skin, deep in the dermal fat about ¼ inch from the surface of the skin. The colors you see are imprinted on the cortex of the hair fibers; the cuticle that covers the hair bundles is clear.

These two pigments affect your hair in the following ways:

✔ **Eumelanin,** the most common pigment, controls black and brown colors (slightly different dominant genes)

✔ **Phaeomelanin** has a red color to it; all humans have some degree of red pigment in their hair, except for people whose hair is stark white

The amount of eumelanin in the hair determines the darkness of the color in the following way:

✔ Brown eumelanin in large quantities will make the hair dark brown.

✔ Brown eumelanin in low quantities will produce a blond color.

✔ Black eumelanin will make the hair black.

✔ Black eumelanin in very low concentrations will create gray hair.

Most hair colors are a balance between brown, black, and red pigment, based upon the amount of these pigments that blend together. Northern Europe has more blond-haired people than anywhere else, and Scotland has the highest redheaded population (up to 10 percent of Scots are redheads). The rest of the human race has dark pigment granules. If you bleach your hair, you oxidize these pigments and they lose their color.

If you have no pigment-producing cells (as happens as some people age), your hair will be white. Albinos have no pigment granules and have white hair — even their eyebrows and eyelashes.

Phaeomelanin is a robust pigment with a strong impact on the hair. It's hard to get hair with a high percentage of phaeomelanin to respond to dyes and bleaches. Salon operators know that when people bleach their hair, their natural red pigment lingers, so it's not unusual for bleached hair to show a red or orange tinge (particularly in blonds) and over time turn orange and various shades of yellow with exposure to light.

How dyes work

Hair dyes can be either permanent or semi-permanent. Both are easy to apply at home, reasonably inexpensive, and very popular, but can also be damaging to your hair, especially if they're not used properly.

Settling for semi-permanent

Semi-permanent dyes are acidic and are made of small molecules that can pass through the scales of the cuticle and into the hair cortex. These dyes are water-soluble and easily washed out. They may last from one to six weeks, depending on what dyes are used, but they lose color faster with frequent washings. Semi-permanent dyes are generally safe and can be used at home. Because they don't contain bleach, they can't lighten hair, but they can darken graying hair.

If you decide you're unhappy with your new semi-permanent color, many home ingredients can help you rinse out the dye. Common hair rinse ingredients found around the house include tea, beer (which is also thought to add body to the hair and make it more manageable), lemon juice, and heavily diluted honey (50 drops in a pint of water). Rinse with any of these remedies after washing your hair if you want the dye out faster. The sooner you wash out the dye, the quicker it will come out.

You may not want to walk around with your hair smelling of beer, so you can follow up the rinse with a more pleasant smelling shampoo.

Going platinum

Bleaches oxidize the melanin granules in the cortex of the hair, causing them to lose their color. This is an irreversible chemical alteration in the hair itself and can't be washed out. The most common bleach for hair is hydrogen peroxide, which can be used in conjunction with dyes to achieve the desired color.

Bleaches are often alkaline solutions, just like the neutralizing solutions used for perms, which open the scales on the cuticle (for more on perms, see the later section, "Perming your hair"). When you bleach dark hair, the small concentrations of phaeomelanin are resistant to the bleach so it's not unusual to see a red tinge on bleached dark hair.

The powerful bleach needed to obtain the platinum blond look will almost certainly damage the hair cuticle, especially if it takes several applications to achieve the desired color, each adding more damage to the cuticle. The hair loses its silky feel because of the cuticle damage.

Bleaching also makes hair more porous, which can produce uneven shading. As new hair grows in its original color at the scalp level, the entire head of hair often must be bleached again to cover it, producing more potential damage to the older part of the hair shaft. Some people just bleach their roots, targeting the hair close to the scalp but leaving the hair that emerges from the scalp in its original color.

With repeated bleaching, wet combing is difficult because the hair cuticle isn't smooth and has many damaged scales. Back combing (or teasing) this hair just compounds the problem, producing mechanical damage and hair breakage as the scales are knocked off. Bleached hair also swells very easily because it's so porous, and hair is much weaker when it's wet.

Putting on permanent coloring

Permanent hair coloring can be applied to the whole head or just in select areas for streaks or highlights. Before hair can be permanently dyed, all the existing color has to be removed by a strong hydrogen peroxide (in a concentration of 30 to 40 percent) that bleaches out all the melanin granules. This may produce some permanent damage to the keratin in the hair cortex, leaving the hair with a lifeless look.

Ammonia is the alkaline chemical applied to open the cuticle and allow the hair color to penetrate the cortex of the hair. It also acts as a catalyst (accelerating the chemical reaction) when the permanent hair color comes together with the peroxide.

Various alcohols and conditioners may also be present in permanent hair color. The conditioners close the scales on the cuticle after coloring in order to seal the new color to the cortex. Closing the scales of the cuticle is important to maintain the moisture of the hair cortex.

The FDA requires that warnings appear on permanent hair color packaging to alert you to possible damage to your hair if directions aren't followed exactly. Read the instructions in the packages carefully.

Perming your hair

Many men and women who are experiencing hair thinning opt for a perm to give their hair a fuller look. You can find more on ways to conceal hair loss in Chapter 8.

Perming your hair correctly is an art. The process is actually quite intricate. Chew on this info when sitting in the salon next time you get a perm!

Permanents use strong alkaline chemicals to break down the disulfide bonds in your hair and open the cortex of the hair fibers within the cuticle so they're able to take on water and reshape themselves anatomically. After the bonds are broken down, the hair can be reformed by using perm rods (the wider the rod, the looser the curl).

Neutralizers that reset your hair in the new curled pattern are applied after rinsing away the setting agent. The neutralizers contain oxidizing agents like hydrogen peroxide, which harden the cement that bonds the hair fibers with its keratin and reform the disulphide bonds to their new shape.

When setting agents are on your hair, your hair is very vulnerable to damage. Changes in the temperature (a person running out of the salon to say hello to someone passing by in the street) can cause damage. The longer the chemicals are in the hair shaft, the more chance there is of damage to the cuticle, and a damaged hair cuticle can leave hair more susceptible to damage from the perming chemicals.

Although the setting agent is washed out before your hair is neutralized, some of the solution will remain in the cortex and continue to have an influence on the hair bundles. For this reason, it's important not to wash your hair for three days after perming, or it may lose the perm prematurely.

Fine hair is more likely to be damaged by repeated perming treatments because the cuticles are thin and the shaft cement and the hair bundles don't contain much bulk for repeated reshaping.

Some people just don't perm well; their hair is resistant to the process, requiring more chemicals and possibly more risks in the perming process. Stronger chemicals increase the risks, so expertise is critical. Permanent damage to the hair and to the growth center below the skin surface increases in probability as stronger chemicals are used to perm or relax the hair. (The next section covers relaxing treatments.)

Relaxing your hair

People with curly or kinky hair use relaxing treatments to make their hair more manageable; it's most common among African Americans or others with unmanageably curly hair. Relaxing is a similar process to perming because the disulphide bond and reforming process in the setting stage is identical, but it's different in that the goal is to straighten the hair, not to curl and shape it. The shape of the hair shaft of the very curly or kinky hair adds a mechanical problem to the straightening process.

Unfortunately, some people are so aggressive with hair straightening chemicals that they do permanent damage to some or all of their hair. Overusing the setting agents can damage the hair above the skin at the hair shaft level or below the skin in the living parts of the hair follicle and cause the hairs to break off. We've seen almost complete permanent hair loss from an overly aggressive use of these setting agents. Damage can be limited by making sure you follow the directions on the use of these chemicals to the letter.

Hot irons may be used in conjunction with relaxing treatments to straighten kinky hair, causing injury to the underlying anatomy of the hair. It's actually easier and less dangerous to straighten very kinky long hair by putting wet hair under a paper bag and using a hot iron on top of the bag. The paper minimizes the damage to the cuticle because it insulates the hair from the high temperatures of the hot iron.

Avoiding Hair Damage

Hair is under constant assault, not only from the elements (sun, wind, and rain) but also from you, its owner. There are endless ways to torture your hair into submission — and in some cases the damage can be permanent. In this section, we look at the things that make your hair cry uncle and things you can do to counteract the damage you may have already inflicted.

Because you're constantly producing new hair, you can get a fresh start, a second chance at caring for your hair if you did things wrong in the recent past. This means that you replace the old damaged hair with new freshly growing hair, but it will take months for this process to occur (hair grows at ½ inch per month). Improper use of permanent dyes or hair setting agents can damage all of the hair on top of your head.

You may have to wait a year or two for new growth to replace that which must be cut away, but the hair will grow back, as long as you haven't inflicted permanent damage on the hair root. The longer you want your hair, the longer the wait.

Hair in thinning areas is often finer than hair on other parts of your head. Thinning hair also grows more slowly. If hair in the frontal or crown areas where hair is starting to miniaturize (the step before it disappears permanently) is damaged in any way, its growth may stop completely until it has time to recover — and at that point, the hair may be about to disappear permanently.

Unfortunately, the period where hair begins to thin is the time people often start trying to make their thinning hair look better by dyeing it. Aggressive dying may finish off the balding process ahead of time.

Most people do dastardly things to their hair on a daily basis; here are just a few of the worst offenses:

- **Drying with a blow-dryer:** Deep in the cortex are air pockets that give hair an added bounce. These air pockets have moisture in them, and if you blow-dry your hair at a high temperature, you can boil the moisture and cause the hair shaft to explode! So a moderate temperature is essential when you blow-dry your hair.

- **Using hot rollers:** These curl-creators may be the single most damaging thing for hair because they apply heat directly to your hair.

- **Exposing hair to direct sunlight:** Heat decreases the amount of moisture in your hair, causing problems similar to those of blow-drying. Exposing your hair to high doses of ultraviolet light from direct sunlight can cause significant damage to the disulphide bonds in the keratin.

- **Rubbing too hard to dry hair:** If you rub your hair roughly with a towel, the friction pulls out hair and may produce mechanical damage to the remaining hair shafts.

✔ **Hacking it with dull scissors:** Dull scissors can split apart the cuticle, leaving broken hair with split ends that tend to peel down the hair shaft.

✔ **Back brushing:** Think of your hair as a one-way street which runs from the scalp to the tip of the hair follicle. When you brush or comb the hair against the scales, going from the tip of the follicle to the scalp, you can irreversibly damage the shaft and break the hair. Intact, unbroken cuticle cells are glossy and smooth and give hair its shine and luster. Back brushing changes the character of the cuticle so that it loses its shine and luster.

✔ **Using a metal comb or brushing too hard:** Plastic combs create much less friction than metal combs and are a better choice. Combing or brushing wet hair can fracture the hair shafts, but conditioners can help by detangling and allowing a comb to be passed through the hair without tugging on it, which may cause it to fracture. When combing, start at the ends and work your way up to the scalp, making sure to stay with the grain by combing downward away from the scalp.

✔ **Perming:** As we explain in the earlier section, "Perming your hair," the perming process breaks apart the scales so that water can be absorbed and the hair can be reshaped. Leaving perm solution on for too long or perming too often can permanently damage the hair shaft.

✔ **Bleaching or coloring:** The earlier section, "How dyes work," explains how bleaching or coloring your hair can damage the cuticle and increase the porosity of the hair shaft, weakening the hair by allowing it to absorb too much moisture.

✔ **Putting rubber bands around it:** Rubber bands can cause traction alopecia by putting too much pressure on the hair shafts. In fact, constant pulling of the hair from any source can cause traction alopecia.

✔ **Using hair sprays:** Hair spray coats the cuticle and changes its porosity, and it makes hairs bind to each other and pull at the points of contact. They can produce traction from the constant pulling that may fracture the hair cuticle and the spindles below, exposing the cortex to possible environmental damage.

Most hair sprays are water-soluble, so if you wash your hair daily after using hair sprays, the hair spray chemicals and bonds they form are usually washed away, decreasing the chance of damage.

An occasional bad hair day doesn't mean you've permanently damaged your hair; bad hair days usually are caused by a reduction in static electricity in your hair, which is due to weather conditions and not by anything you've done to your hair.

You guarantee that your hair will recover poorly from damage from the various hair treatments you subject it to if you don't give it an opportunity for repair with good washing and conditioning. Once the cuticle cracks or breaks and the cortex is damaged, only a good hair cut (removing the damaged hair by cutting it off) will allow you to get the healthy hair look you want.

 When hair is damaged, it appears dull and feels rough, losing that silky feel. Fortunately, with time, the hair grows out and you can cut away that damaged hair as the younger part of the hair near the base of the scalp replaces the old hair.

Maintaining a Healthy Scalp

There's a common misconception that balding means there's something wrong with the scalp. But because hair actually starts growing from below the scalp, the scalp itself has little to do with hair loss or hair health.

When hair loss occurs because of male genetic hair loss (or any other cause), the blood supply to the area drops because it isn't needed where there isn't any hair. When surgeons transplant new hair, the circulation in the scalp improves as the new hair grows out (in effect recruiting the blood supply it needs). (You can find more about hair transplantation in Part V.)

We generally tell patients that if they shampoo with a good commercial product and use a conditioner once a day, the skin of the scalp should remain moist and well taken care of.

You can impact your scalp circulation in a number of ways, some of which may affect your hair indirectly. Things that are bad for the scalp and its circulation include:

- ✔ **Smoking:** As shown in ultrasound studies, smoking reduces scalp circulation. Because this occurs with each cigarette, over time smoking may contribute to whatever hair loss is occurring on the head. Most doctors strongly believe this connection, although definitive scientific proof is lacking.

- ✔ **Sun exposure:** Repeated sunburns on the scalp may impact structures deep in the scalp causing the hair producing cells to shrink. Combining genetic hair loss and intense ultraviolet light may speed up the balding process.

- ✔ **Skin cancer:** Skin cancer comes in three different types, two of which can be deadly by spreading throughout your body (malignant melanomas and squamous cell cancers). These cancers almost always appear in sun exposed skin.

Melanomas can rapidly spread beyond the confines of the local area and they can be very small flat, mole like, frequently black tumors. The third type of cancer, basal cell cancer) usually remains local but it often produces ulcers on the skin, and they can grow to a significant size.

When balding occurs, the scalp is exposed to the impact of ultraviolet light from direct sunlight, and the skin changes from a smooth, uniform colored skin, to a skin that has spots and discolorations throughout. Hair protects the scalp from direct sunlight and can produce enough shade to reduce the risks of skin cancers.

✔ **Dermatologic conditions:** A variety of conditions can impact the skin and scalp. See Chapter 5 for more.

✔ **Folliculitis:** This is an infection of the hair follicles. It appears as acne or red or white bumps on the scalp skin and may have to be treated with soaks, antibiotics, or a minor surgical incision. It should never be picked or scratched, as this may increase the incidence of permanent scarring and may spread the infection from an infected hair follicle to one that is not infected.

Folliculitis rarely causes permanent hair loss, but it may cause the hair to prematurely enter the telogen (sleep) phase of the hair cycle.

✔ **Chlorine and salt water:** Frequent swimming in chlorine pools or salt water without shampooing and conditioning afterward has the ability to cause hair and scalp damage from the heavy salt or chlorine exposure. The salt can dry the scalp.

Many patients believe that dandruff may cause balding, but this is not true. Other patients report having an itchy or tingling scalp, and they believe it's a precursor of the balding process. This complaint is actually quite common and may be a sign of early genetic hair loss.

Caring for Children's Hair

Want to get a head start on healthy heads of hair for your kids? You can do this by teaching them how to properly wash and dry their hair. Help them learn non-destructive styling techniques (until they reach the age where their friends know way more than you do about hair — and everything else).

Many babies have little hair to work with, and what hair they have is often very fine, delicate, and easily damaged. As a child grows, new hair grows that's often thicker than the baby hairs seen in the first year of life.

In many infants, the new hair grown at about one year may have a completely different texture or color than what was previously present!

Probably the most damage to children's hair comes from the styles used to make them look cute or to keep their hair out of their faces! Ponytails, pigtails, and braids can pull out the hair at the roots and produce traction alopecia (see Chapter 5 for more on traction alopecia). This hair loss condition is very common among African American children, who often have multiple pigtails that pull on the scalp in many areas, or Caucasian children with wild or very curly hair. Unfortunately, this type of hair loss is often permanent.

People take so much pride in the way their children look that they often treat the kids like dolls, using hairstyles that are counter to the hair's natural growing tendencies and that can harm the hair over time. To avoid damaging a young person's hair, follow these recommendations (most of the rules discussed earlier in this chapter apply just as much to children as they do to adults):

- ✔ **Don't keep rubber bands in the hair overnight.**

- ✔ **Rotate hairstyles so that one area isn't always receiving traction.** For example, do a ponytail one day, braids the next, and then leave it loose with a headband for a day or two.

- ✔ **Use a good conditioner to make the hair slide more easily when you're combing out knots.** For longer hair, use detangling agents along with a good conditioner to minimize the formation of knots in the first place.

  As with adult hair, always start at the end of the hair and work toward the scalp, not the other direction. (Hardly anyone does this properly, but now you know!)

  When working on knots, hold the hair between the ends and the scalp tightly in one hand as you comb the hair so that the child doesn't feel the pain of the comb pulling on the hair.

- ✔ **Use a plastic comb rather than a brush to prevent static electricity from building on the hair as it dries.** Static electricity will make the hair stand up with more exposure to the elements like sun, heat, and wind.

- ✔ **Never back comb the hair, as this is guaranteed to damage children's delicate hair shafts.**

- ✔ **Encourage children's involvement in hair care.** Show them how to properly wash and dry their hair and comb out tangles, and help them choose a flattering and easy care hairstyle.

Fostering independence in proper hair grooming should be your goal.

✔ **Inspect your children's hair on a regular basis, especially when they start school.** Hair lice is practically a rite of passage for school-aged children and is easily spread from child to child. Early detection and treatment is important in minimizing any effects that head lice can have on the hair, such as permanent patches of hair loss.

✔ **Make hair care fun.** Hair care should be an enjoyable experience.

Get off to a good start by using no-tears shampoos and patting hair dry to eliminate the pain and suffering of hair washing. Play with suds, styling dramatic and funny do's.

Managing your children's hair gives you an opportunity to share an important common experience. Throughout your children's lives, hair will be important, and if you use their hair to help instill pride in their looks, you help enhance their self-esteem.

Part II

The Root of Hair Loss: How and Why It Happens

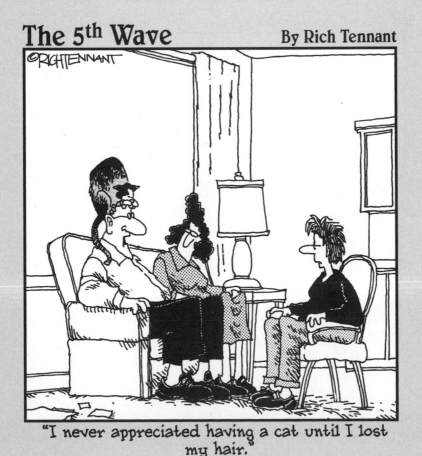

"I never appreciated having a cat until I lost my hair."

In this part . . .

All hair loss isn't the same. People lose hair due to hereditary factors, illnesses, and a number of other reasons. In this section, we look at how and why hair loss occurs as well as what you can do to prevent it.

Chapter 4

Types of Hair Loss and Pattern Thinning in Men and Women

- -

In This Chapter

▶ Defining the various types of hair loss

▶ Understanding how heredity and disease can cause hair loss

▶ Looking at how your lifestyle impacts your hair

▶ Exploring causes of pattern thinning in men and women

- -

*P*eople have different ideas about what constitutes hair loss and what causes it. Some people see three or four hairs in the sink after combing and panic. Others don't think they're losing their hair until the back bald spot meets the middle bald spot and there's nothing left to comb. When it comes to figuring out why they're going bald, some people assume it's genetic, and therefore unavoidable, whereas others are less accepting and look into every possible way to save their hair.

In this chapter, we define male and female balding patterns, explain why balding occurs, describe how pattern baldness is recognized and classified, and give you some ideas on how your lifestyle can affect your hair.

Defining Different Types of Hair Loss

How do you define hair loss? Do you consider you're balding when you've lost 5 hairs, 5,000, or 50,000? Can you slow the balding process, stop it altogether, or should you just increase your baseball hat collection and live with it?

Hair falls out of your head every single day, at a rate of about 100 to 150 hairs if you are a Caucasian (Asians lose 80–120 per day and Africans 60–100 per day). You aren't going bald if your hair is coming out at these rates because that is the rate that new hair grows up from the scalp. If the hair that falls out isn't replaced by the same number of new hairs, then you have a balding problem. Hair loss isn't noticeable in the average person until more than 50 percent is lost, which is around 50,000 hairs, more or less.

Why does hair loss occur at all? You were born with your hair, and by simple logic, you should die with it, right? Not one organ in the human body dies as a natural course of aging, yet hair follicles commit mass suicide over time. Other human organs may change over time and become less functional, but they don't disappear altogether. Is hair loss a type of genetic adaptation? No one knows.

This section looks at the different types and causes of hair loss, including the cause of 99 percent of all cases of male balding: male pattern baldness.

Telling the difference between genetic baldness and everything else

There's more than one category of hair loss. Can your doctor tell just by looking at you what kind of hair loss you have? Yes, sometimes. Hereditary hair loss patterns, the most common type of hair loss in men, have developed into a classical clinical descriptive science. Genetic hair loss appears in distinct patterns, and these patterns are almost 100-percent diagnostic for male pattern baldness. The later section, "Norwood classifications for measuring male pattern thinning" covers the most common baldness patterns. Also, we discuss the types and causes of pattern balding in the later section, "Common Causes of Hair Loss."

In women, balding patterns also exist (see the section, "Genetic hair loss in women," later in this chapter), and a knowledgeable doctor may be able to tell what's causing the hair loss just by looking.

Examining uniform hair loss

A small segment of people lose scalp hair uniformly (diffusely), rather than losing hair in specific scalp areas. Uniform hair loss isn't as easy to detect as other types of hair loss because the hair is steadily lost all over the head. It's much easier to detect a bald spot resulting from hair loss in a specific area of the scalp from diseases that cause uniform hair loss to the normal genetics of that particular person.

Hair loss occurs normally and usually occurs at the end of one of the normal hair cycles that all hair goes through. These hair cycles are as follows:

- **Anagen:** The growth stage, which lasts three years on average but may be as short as a year and as long as seven years).

- **Catogen:** The stage when the hair prepares to go into the next phase and undergoes changes in its anatomy, falling out at the end of this part of the cycle.

- **Telogen:** The sleep phase when a percentage of the hair disappears (lasts from two to five months on average). About 10 percent of all of the hairs on our head are in the telogen part of the cycle at any one time.

At the end of the telogen phase, a new hair bud appears, signaling the beginning of anagen. (Chapter 2 has more about hair growth phases.)

The hair apparatus starts off producing a baby hair below the skin, which grows longer and longer until the final *terminal hair* (a full mature hair reflective of what we style every day when we comb out hair) emerges from the pore in the skin. In some adults, the anagen phase may never start, signaling that the hair follicle may have died. If a new hair doesn't grow to replace the lost hair, the total hair count drops.

Hair grows in natural occurring groups called *follicular units* (FU). A single FU contains from one to four terminal hairs and one *vellus hair* (a fine hair amidst the clump of terminal hairs). When a hair isn't replaced after its telogen phase, the number of hairs in the FU decreases, but the number of FUs remains the same. So an FU starting with four terminal hairs may end up with only two or three terminal hairs as we age or as we undergo some form of balding. When this happens across the whole scalp, the total hair count decreases proportionally.

The older the patient is, the more likely it is that doctors see this uniform hair loss process. About one third of men over age 70 have this diffuse hair loss, which is called *senile alopecia*. The name doesn't reflect the mental status of those afflicted, but rather it essentially means that the condition is most common in the elderly. Because hair also becomes finer with age, severe thinning reflects a loss of both hair bulk (in each hair shaft) and hair densities. (For more on hair bulk and density, turn to Chapter 2.) There's no cure for senile alopecia.

Young men may experience uniform hair loss in the form of a condition called *diffuse unpatterned alopecia* (DUPA). Doctors believe that DUPA and senile alopecia are similar but for the age of occurrence. DUPA impacts men in their 20s and 30s and doesn't seem to be responsive to drugs used to treat the classic type of male patterned hair loss. We cover treatment drugs in Chapter 9.

Identifying dying hair cells

Apoptosis is a cell's internal "suicide" mechanism that causes cell death. The phenomenon has recently been studied very carefully, and what doctors know is that during the transition from anagen to catagen (that's the growth phase to the changing phase), something happens in the hair follicle development.

The cells within the hair follicles communicate with each other, and certain chemicals secreted in the hair follicle determine which hairs will survive for another growth cycle and which will die. Experts believe that the lifespan of each hair follicle — and possibly each follicular unit — is genetically programmed.

Because some of the hair follicles within the FU survive while others die, there's some hope that the chemical inducers that determine the survivors can be identified and manipulated to prevent hair loss. We have identified some of the molecules that stimulate the process but others still need to be isolated. Maybe when all of the molecules are identified and isolated, we can stop the balding process from occurring.

Saving dying hair cells

The causes of cell death are complex. Research has shown that the cells that produce apoptosis-causing chemicals are found in every part of the hair follicle. It's possible that different types of hair loss are influenced by different chemical problems in the pathways that control cell death.

Although the medical community is identifying many of these chemical pathways, it's no closer to finding a cure for apoptosis than we would like. Interestingly, apoptosis typically doesn't occur in cancerous cells, which are thought to be immortal, escaping their natural destiny of living a given number of cell cycles. For example, in breast cancer, a gene called BRCA causes the production of a particular enzyme that blocks apoptosis. Imagine if it were possible to bottle that enzyme to use on hair that's dying off or, even better, create a cocktail that could make all the cells in the body immortal! At least we can dream.

Common Causes of Hair Loss

A number of diseases and conditions cause hair loss, but most people go bald because of the influence of genetics, hormones, and time. Stress may cause additional loss, more so in women than in men.

Looking at Grandpa's head

In the genetic hair loss lottery, Grandpa's important, but doctors actually look a few generations back on the entire family tree — men and women — in order to determine if you've inherited a genetic type of pattern baldness.

 Everyone inherits genetic tendencies from their parents. As you may or may not recall from biology class, pairs of DNA segments called *chromosomes* carry the information that contains the potential for different characteristics. A *gene* is a single bit of chemically encoded hereditary instruction located on a chromosome.

The genetics of *androgenetic alopecia* (ANA), also called *androgenetic alopecia* or *male pattern baldness,* is complicated. At least four genes are responsible for hair loss. When several genes need to be present for a trait such as hair loss, the trait is said to be *polygenic.* Genes that are located on the X or Y chromosomes are called *sex-linked,* and genes on the other 22 pairs of chromosomes are called *autosomal.*

Currently, doctors believe that the genes governing common baldness are autosomal (not tied to the sex chromosome) and therefore can be inherited from the mother's or the father's side of the family. The commonly held notion that baldness comes only from the mother's side of the family is false, although for reasons not fully understood, the predisposition inherited from an affected mother is of slightly greater importance than that inherited from an affected father. Doctors also believe that the genes involved in androgenetic alopecia are *dominant,* meaning that only one gene of a pair is needed for the trait to show up in the individual. So even if only one of your parents passed on the baldness gene, you're likely to have some hair loss.

 The inherited gene isn't always 'expressed,' so it's possible to carry the gene for balding and never become bald. It can skip a generation or two, so only looking at the generation before you doesn't tell you what may happen on *your* head.

The ability of a gene to affect you is called *expressivity.* Expressivity occurs depending on a number of factors, the major ones being hormones and age, although stress and other factors may also play a role. Put simply, a man whose father and uncles are severely bald may have minimal hair loss because the expression of the baldness gene is limited. If you are confused by this explanation, imagine the experts who try to clarify the unexplainable by putting together the many variables and not coming up with a logical, scientific process.

The end goal of gene identification is to manipulate genes to prevent or reverse common baldness. But doctors first need to find and fully understand which genes cause the balding process and why are these genes expressed one way in you and another way in your brother.

Hormonal influences on hair

Hormones are very powerful biochemical substances produced by various glands throughout the body. The primary male sex hormone is testosterone. Testosterone and other related hormones that have "masculinizing" effects are produced primarily in the testicles. These same hormones are the cause of many changes that occur in puberty in boys. The hormones that cause acne and beard growth also can trigger the beginning of baldness. Testosterone is also produced in women from the adrenal glands and the ovaries, and it is produced in lower concentrations than the testicles produce the hormone in men. In women, most of the testosterone is converted into estrogen.

The hormone believed to be most directly involved in androgenetic alopecia is *dihydrotestosterone* (DHT). DHT is formed by the action of the enzyme 5-alpha reductase (5AR) on testosterone, and it binds to special receptor sites on the cells of hair follicles to cause the specific changes associated with balding.

The presence of androgens (steroid like substances), testosterone (considered an androgen), and DHT cause some hair follicles to regress and die. In addition to the testicles, the adrenal glands located above the kidneys produce androgenetic hormones; this is true for both sexes. In females, ovaries are the major source of hormones that can affect hair. Androgenetic hormones stimulate many of the male sex characteristics we see in adult men. Androgens like testosterone, are converted into estrogens in women, which make women develop their typical female sex characteristics.

Baring hair at the beach

The beach is an excellent place to observe hair patterns. Have you ever noticed that men with hairy backs and shoulders often have a bald head or a hair replacement system?

This indicates that the gene for hair on the back and shoulders is separate from the gene for hair on the scalp. Although DHT acts like fertilizer for shoulder and back hair, it causes reduction of head hair in many men.

Early in the 20th century, a psychiatrist discovered the specific relationship between testosterone and hormone-induced hair loss. The doctor noted that the identical twin brother of one patient was profoundly bald while the mentally ill twin had a full head of hair. The doctor decided to determine the effect of treating his patient with testosterone, and injected him (the hairy twin) with the hormone. Within weeks, the hairy patient began to lose all but his wreath of permanent hair, just like his twin. The doctor stopped administering testosterone, but his patient never regained his head of hair.

Testosterone and DHT

The cause of pattern thinning in men is primarily related to two sex hormones, testosterone and DHT. The body converts testosterone into the hormone DHT by way of an enzyme found in various tissues throughout the body.

In men with the genes for ANA, DHT increases the resting (telogen) phase and decreases the growing (anagen) phase of hair. (We explain the growth cycle more in the earlier section, "Examining uniform hair loss.") Consequently, as a man ages, less hair grows at any given time, and the hair starts to thin as a normal consequence of aging, especially in men with ANA. Eventually, baldness occurs. In men who haven't inherited the ANA balding genes, the combination of DHT and testosterone doesn't cause hair loss and may have a lesser impact on aging hair.

Some areas of the scalp are more susceptible than others to the affects of DHT. For example, the hormone doesn't usually affect hair on the back and side of the head, which is why these areas retain hair. The term "male pattern thinning" is used because hair loss occurs in a pattern — the back and side of the head retain hair but the crown and frontal areas may lose it. The loss may be confined only to the frontal area or the crown area based upon the genetics that are inherited from the family tree.

DHT does play a role in the growth of beard hair; body hair; and eyebrow, nose, and ear hair, but doctors don't clearly understand that role. Sometime after puberty, male hormones trigger a biological clock that makes hair grow in these areas.

In men, the enzyme 5AR activity is higher in the balding area. Women have half the amount of 5AR overall as compared to men but have higher levels of the enzyme aromatase, especially in their frontal hairlines. Aromatase decreases the formation of DHT, and its presence in women may help to explain why female hair loss is somewhat different than hair loss in males. (The section "Examining Hair Thinning in Women" later in this chapter takes an in-depth look at female hair loss.)

The only way to stop DHT is to block it with *finasteride* or *dutasteride,* drugs that interfere with DHT production. (See Chapter 9 for more on DHT and the drugs that fight hair loss.)

 At present, only finasteride has been approved by the Federal Drug Administration (FDA). Dutasteride is still being evaluated for its safety and effectiveness for hair loss in young men. There are some reports that dutasteride has significant effects on male sperm production; as such, it may not be approved for men experiencing hair loss. Blocking DHT in women with dutasteride hasn't been shown to prevent or reverse female hair loss or hair thinning. Its safety with regard to breast cancer, particularly in women who carry the breast cancer producing BRCA genes, is not understood.

Steroids and similar products

Anabolic steroids, the kind bodybuilders sometimes (illegally) use, can cause hair loss if you're genetically predisposed to it. And there's a direct link between taking human growth hormone (HGH) and hair loss — probably caused by the same underlying mechanisms as steroid use. Women body builders who take steroids develop some male sex characteristics and some experience hair loss.

 HGH has become a trendy anti-aging tool. More and more men are using it as a fountain of youth. Some men combine steroids and HGH because they make them feel better and stronger. But we have seen many men on HGH in our offices with "unexplained hair loss." No real mystery there.

Many men who take steroids also take Propecia (a DHT blocker) to offset the negative effects of DHT. Propecia blocks DHT and causes a rise in systemic testosterone by up to 18 percent. Indirectly, Propecia may help muscle building if DHT levels go down (from the Propecia) and testosterone levels go up to compensate.

Testosterone is a much stronger hormone than DHT, and the sum of the effects of the rise in serum testosterone from taking a DHT blocker such as Propecia and the steroids may very well produce more hair loss, not less.

Everyone is different, so we can't conclude if the muscle mass that the men are seeking from steroid use can be offset. Recently, Propecia was found to mask the blood measurements for other steroids when used in athletes, which is why its use is banned for professional athletes.

Fitness-focused individuals may take the following products for their physical benefits, but these products can also cause hair loss:

- ✔ **Whey-based nutritional supplements:** The use of growth hormones in some dairy cows affects the milk they produce and, in turn, the whey (a byproduct of cheese production). Even if a person doesn't take steroids, these products may have some steroid-like impact from the milk source. People who take whey-based nutritional supplements may experience steroid-related side effects if the cows were treated with steroids. It is unclear how much of these steroids, if any, will survive transit through the stomach to be eventually absorbed into the body.

- ✔ **DHEA:** Some people take DHEA, which is found in the nutritional section of many health food and vitamin stores and doesn't require a prescription. The DHEA sold in stores is reportedly made by the adrenal glands and claims to help reduce body fat stores while promoting sugar metabolism. It also can cause hair loss. Other available supplements claim testosterone or steroid-like characteristics. The desire for men to add body mass and/or prevent hair loss drives them to seek out such products.

- ✔ **Dose-pack steroids:** A short course of steroids for medical reasons (4–5 days) should not have an impact producing hair loss.

- ✔ **Prednisone:** People who are on this steroid for chronic medical problems (arthritis, various autoimmune diseases) will experience hair loss.

Hair loss is also a risk for women who use steroids, if they're predisposed to the condition. Women usually take steroids for diseases that occur later in life, such as autoimmune disease, temporal arteritis, rheumatoid arthritis.

Hair loss over time

The mere presence of the necessary genes and hormones for hair loss isn't enough to cause baldness. Susceptible hair follicles also have to be exposed to the responsible hormones. The onset of hair loss varies from one individual to another and is influenced by genetic expression, the levels of testosterone and DHT in the bloodstream, and age.

Hair loss doesn't occur all at once, but is cyclical. People who are losing their hair experience alternating periods of slow hair loss and rapid hair loss, and even periods when hair loss stabilizes. The factors that cause the rate of loss to speed up or slow down are unknown.

Most men who have extensive balding develop much of it by age 30. Twenty-five percent of men will show clinical balding by age 30, and half of the male population will show some degree of clinical balding by age 45 to 50. Balding slowly continues into the next decade or two, and then the process seems to slow down as men approach 60 to 65. As this is a genetic process, it is probable that the men who bald later in life rather than earlier also have a form of genetic hair loss, just not the obvious process we see in the younger men with classic pattern balding.

Men who continue the balding process well into their 30s and 40s typically don't lose their hair as quickly or as completely as men who start balding in their early 20s. About 7 percent of men who are balding develop the most complete form of balding (called the Class VII pattern; see Figure 4-1), in which only the wreath of hair exists around the head. Those men with Class VII balding patterns, usually show those patterns before they reach 30 years old. This wreath of hair is permanent hair in most men and measures about 2½ inches in the mid-back of the head when the balding process reaches completion. Most men who show balding don't advance to full balding.

To make matters more confusing, the age of onset discussed above reflects the majority of men, yet there are still some men who start the process later in life (in their 30s, 40s, and even 50s).

The most common balding patterns are seen at the frontal hairline where frontal and temporal recession occurs, moving slightly upward toward the top of the head. A bald spot may appear in the crown and when it does, it seems to widen slowly as men age. Sometimes, the crown balding area merges with the frontal recession, clearing a wide bald channel in the center of the head that we jokingly call the "runway." Genetics determine the final pattern.

Stress

When the body experiences stress caused by a traumatic experience, nutritional deficiency, or illness, the rate of hair loss can
increase. For example, a 39-year-old patient of Dr. Rassman lost his
4-year-old child to cancer and within just a few months, the man lost
all but the permanent wreath of hair around his head. He probably
had the genetics for this balding pattern, but only expressed that
pattern when it was induced by this extreme stressful situation.

Women's hair seems to be more sensitive to the effects of stress
than men's hair. This may be because women with a genetic predisposition to hair loss usually have a higher percentage of fragile
miniaturized hair, which is hair with thinner than normal hair shaft
thickness. But unlike in men, the hair loss in women is often not
permanent or complete.

Stress generally causes a type of hair loss referred to as *telogen
effluvium,* which is very different from androgenetic alopecia (discussed earlier in this chapter). Telogen effluvium is the reversible
shedding of hair in the resting phase when the body senses, for
reasons that are not clear, that it needs to divert its energies.
Therefore, stress temporarily changes the amount of hair that's
shed, but the lost hair is likely to grow back. Turn to Chapter 5 for
more explanation of telogen effluvium.

Lack of blood supply

Some doctors assert that a lack of blood supply contributes to hair
loss. Bald skin gradually loses some of its blood supply and as a
result becomes thin and shiny. These changes, however, come only
after the loss of hair and is not the cause of the hair loss.

Hair follicles are some of the most rapidly metabolizing cells in the
body. Growing hair requires the proper oxygen and nutrition that
comes with a good blood supply in a healthy body. When hair follicles are transplanted into skin grafts or scar tissue, both of which
may have a relatively poor blood supply, the presence of the
grafted hair causes the local blood supply to increase. The end
result is that as the hair grows, so does the blood supply.

Environmental issues

Can you eat yourself into a full head of hair? Probably not, but environmental factors, including what you eat, can cause hair loss. The
following list breaks down some of the more prominent factors:

- ✔ **Selenium:** The presence of selenium in food and water is common around the world, but continued intake of selenium to the point of selenium toxicity produces hair loss, among other effects.

- ✔ **Lead, cadmium, mercury, iron, aluminum, and copper:** These are the most common environmental causes of hair loss. Many of these substances are found in fish, reflecting environmental contamination in the world's oceans. Lead may also be found in hair dyes and paint. Just how much of these elements must be present to cause hair loss is unknown, and a direct connection is hard to prove. Some labs will analyze hair for the presence of these minerals, but their presence doesn't necessarily mean they caused hair loss.

- ✔ **Air pollution and smoking:** These factors may also exacerbate the genetic process carried by potentially balding men. Scientists believe toxins and carcinogens found in polluted air can stop hair growing by blocking the mechanisms that produce the protein from which hair is made.

Doctors hope that science will discover ways to treat pollutant contributions to hair loss with topical lotions to block the effects of the pollutants on the hair follicles.

Looking at Male Pattern Thinning

Pattern thinning is a specific kind of hair loss that occurs gradually over time. Both men and women can experience pattern thinning, but they experience it differently. In men, pattern thinning sometimes goes by the scientific name *androgenetic alopecia* (ANA). You hear a lot about ANA, as it's the most common reason for hair loss in men. Easily 98 percent of men who are balding have ANA.

Men with ANA usually first notice a thinning or receding hairline in the front at a fairly young age. The pattern progresses to thinning on the crown of the head that may slowly thin over a decade or more. The pattern thinning process tends to begin during early or mid-20s, possibly with some thinning in the teen years, but until the thinning reduces the hair density by 50 percent most of it goes unnoticed.

For the man with patterned hair loss, general areas thin but may not become completely bald initially. Over many years, the hair loss can progress to complete balding, but it's also possible that total loss of hair may not occur.

Male hair loss starts when hair shafts grow thinner in a process called *miniaturization*. As fewer hairs remain after shedding starts, men notice, especially in bright light, that their hair has a "see-through" look. They generally start off denying what they are seeing, and then eventually panic sets in.

Early evidence of pattern thinning

Because male pattern thinning is a genetic condition, a man who comes from a family with many bald members is more likely to be on the lookout for baldness symptoms than a man from a family with full heads of hair. However, because of the nature of ANA, genetics can play tricks on men.

In some families, balding isn't transmitted to the offspring, while in families with full heads of hair, the genes for balding may lie dormant in one generation and then just appear in the next. All too often, a young man can't believe that he's balding because he can't find relatives on either side of the family with balding; the reverse is also true — a man with a full head of hair may see extensive balding in his family line. It's just a role of the genetic dice, we suspect.

Nine out of ten times, men first discover that they're shedding when their shower or bathtub drains get clogged with hair. Regardless of details of the discovery, they may adopt a different hairstyle to cover the signs of hair loss. Some men may abandon combing their hair straight back and adopt a side-to-side combing style that more easily hides thinning hair, continuing this sleight of hand to a point when even this style doesn't cut it. Some men just comb their hair forward so that no one can see what's happening to the front of the head. Look at Rudolf Giuliani and John McCain, who use comb-overs as their slight of hand that is not as slight as they think.

Some men are all too aware of their family's balding problem. They may have teased their father or older brothers about their balding, but it's not so funny when it happens to them.

Those who look for signs of balding or thinning have the opportunity to catch it early. Despite the drug company Merck's promotion of Propecia, many men are unaware that hair loss can be slowed, stopped, or possibly reversed if they take this drug early enough in the pattern thinning process. Treatment can be very successful if the diagnosis is made when the hair loss first become evident, hopefully before substantial thinning has occurred.

The only way to determine if you're at the very beginning of the balding process is to get your hair and scalp mapped out for miniaturization, which is always present when the balding process starts. Mapping requires the use of a video microscope, which examines the hairs all over your head for miniaturization.

As experts in this field, we believe very strongly that if a man is concerned that he may develop hair loss, he should see a doctor to map the scalp hair for the frequency and distribution of miniaturized hairs. Even early pattern thinning corresponds to the balding patterns seen in the Norwood Classification Chart (see Figure 4-1), so doctors can predict the eventual hair loss pattern early on. Annual scalp hair mapping can detect the earliest signs of genetic hair loss before balding can be detected by the naked eye. It can also follow the benefits or lack thereof, of the treatments for balding.

For men, the drug Propecia can be effective at stopping the balding process or at least slowing it down. Unfortunately for women, there's no comparable drug other than Minoxidil, which works only in a small percentage of women.

Norwood classifications for measuring male pattern thinning

Most people think that bald is just plain bald, but doctors measure male pattern thinning by degrees using the Norwood classification system. Dr. O'Tar Norwood devised this classification system in the 1970s, answering the all-important question, "How bald am I?"

Norwood provides two classification systems, one for regular male pattern thinning and one for Type A pattern thinning.

Regular male pattern thinning

Figure 4-1 shows the Norwood classification system for regular male pattern thinning. Under the regular classifications, hair loss is divided into seven patterns. Men may progress from one pattern to the next, or they may develop any one of these patterns all at once as the hair in that pattern thins to complete baldness in the pattern identified on the chart.

The majority of men with pattern thinning follow the regular pattern, with hair loss starting in the front and progressing slowly (front and back) in two different areas (Class IV and V). On rare occasions, a man may just bald in the crown with minimal frontal balding (Class III Vertex). Over time, the frontal and crown areas enlarge and merge, and the entire front, top, and crown of the head may become bald (Class VI or VII).

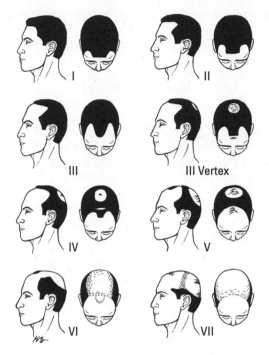

Figure 4-1: Norwood's classification of regular male pattern thinning.

Baldness in some men progresses such that they fall somewhere between the different stages; in other men, hair loss comes to a halt, and they remain in one stage without progressing to the next. Although there's no general agreement on the statistics for the frequency of balding, it's believed that advanced balding (defined as a Norwood Class V, VI, or VII pattern) occurs in about 35 percent of balding men.

In 95 percent of men, the ½ inch of hair on the front of the forehead is lost in the younger years, and the hairline recedes into a *mature male hairline* (somewhere between a Class II or III pattern) with a characteristic convex V-shape. This change from the concave juvenile hairline (also a typical female pattern hairline) to the convex mature male hairline is common and not necessarily a sign of oncoming baldness.

Balding starts at Class III in the Norwood regular classification system (see Figure 4-1). The juvenile hairline is found in all prepubertal boys, whereas a mature hairline appears in 95 percent of Caucasian men ages 18 to 29.

Here's an easy test to find out if your hairline is in its mature position: Lift your eyebrows high and check the distance between the highest crease on your forehead (in the middle) and the beginning of your hairline:

✔ **If your hairline touches the highest crease,** it's in the juvenile position.

✔ **If your hairline is ⅓ to ⅔ inch away from the highest crease,** it's a mature male hairline.

✔ **If your hairline is more than ⅔ inch from the highest crease,** you have frontal balding.

A very small percentage of men keep their juvenile hairlines for many years (former Presidents Ronald Reagan and Bill Clinton are examples of the lucky few). Some men have a *persistent forelock,* thick hair at the central front of the forehead that remains despite pattern thinning or balding around it — like an oasis in the desert (talk-show host David Letterman is one example). The frontal forelock doesn't appear to be subject to the ravages of DHT (refer to the earlier section, "Hormonal influences on hair" for an explanation of DHT), and the frontal hair tends to retain its thickness much like the hair on the sides and back of the head.

Unusual genetics: There appears to be a different genetics in some parts of the head in some people. The ⅔rd inch of the juvenile hairline and the frontal forelock have, in some people, genetics that do not reflect the rest of the frontal part of the head. On rare occasions, we have seen men lose all of their hair in front and on the top except for the frontal ⅔rd inch of hair (just as they had it at the age of 12). This pattern looks strange and each man that presented with this unique pattern of balding tended to exploit the frontal ⅔rd inch by letting it grow out 6–10 inches in length to comb back over their balding head.

Type A pattern thinning

The set of figures in Figure 4-2 shows Type A pattern thinning. Type A thinning is less common than the regular pattern covered in the preceding section, occurring in less than 10 percent of men. In this pattern, hair loss progresses from the front to the back, possibly reaching the crown of the head and stopping about where the swirl exists. Type A pattern thinning is most dramatic in front, and for that reason, Type A men tend to look quite bald even though their hair loss is minimal. Actor Gene Hackman showed the Class A pattern balding for most of his career, and as one followed him in films, his balding pattern creeped from front to back in the classic A pattern.

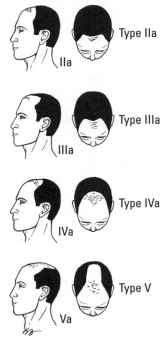

Type IIa

Type IIIa

Type IVa

Type V

Figure 4-2: Type A pattern thinning.

Evolutionary theories for male pattern baldness

Can male pattern baldness be explained by sexual selection? In other words, are males programmed to go bald in order to attract females? Scientists have suggested that, in primitive societies, an enlarged forehead may have conveyed increased maturity and social status — traits that historically have made men more attractive to women.

In *Sex, Time, and Power: How Women's Sexuality Shaped Human Evolution,* (2004), author Leonard Shlain suggests that bald men made the best hunters in primitive, hunter-gatherer societies. Thanks to their lack of hair, bald men could peer over the bush and spy game animals without the animals' recognizing them as men and fleeing. Being better hunters, the bald men were better providers, which made them more attractive to women.

This theory is certainly something to think about when you notice your hair thinning: Women may instinctively like it more than you think.

Examining Hair Thinning in Women

Women are generally more attentive to the appearance of their hair and notice the see-through quality of thinning hair early on. Most women with thinning hair don't lose enough all at once to clog the drain, so problems with styling may be the first sign of the female genetic balding process. This is fortunate because the slow onset of thinning allows women to adjust their styling to compensate for their hair loss.

Most women are able to conceal thinning with a new hairstyle, up to a point. Layering, a pulled-back style like a pony tail, or a bun can hide thinning hair fairly well. Or women can use hair extensions or other hair systems, which we discuss in Chapters 6 and 7.

Regardless of how well they may be able to hide it, hair loss is a psychological challenge for women who fondly remember the luscious, thick hair of their youth and see it coming out in bunches on their hairbrushes. Thinning hair can make a woman feel older and less sexy.

This section looks at genetic female pattern hair loss and other causes of women's hair loss.

Differentiating between possible causes

There are a number of types of identifiable hair loss in women, and they differ based on their causes. The cause of female hair loss is reflected in the pattern, so doctors look to the pattern of loss to get an idea of the cause and how to treat it.

About 10 percent of women experience the classic pattern of genetic hair loss, which is an intact frontal hairline for the first ⅔ inch or so and hair loss behind that persistent hairline. Another recognizable pattern of genetic hair loss in women is hair loss confined to the top of the head, sparing the leading frontal edge of the hair line. Some women with genetic hair loss experience a diffuse hair loss, which is a thinning of the hair all over the head (including the sides and back of the head) and isn't confined to any particular area. This is more common in postmenopausal women, although it does show up in younger women as well.

Perimenopausal women frequently experience pattern thinning that's usually worse in the front of the thinning area, about 2 to 3 inches behind the hairline. Over time, it progresses as far back as the swirl (the place in the crown where hair changes direction and produces a vortex); the thinning areas may spare the sides and back of the head. For perimenopausal women, thinning tends to be diagnosed in the 30s or 40s. It is present but less frequent with women in the 20s. The good news is that once the thinning is recognized in these women it is generally stable over time and does not show the progressive nature of the male balding patterns, at least until they reach menopause.

On the other hand, an advanced presentation of uniform hair loss, called *diffuse unpatterned alopecia* (DUPA), leads doctors to narrow the type of hair loss down to a few distinct possibilities, including female genetic hair loss or senile alopecia.

 Generalized thinning isn't always genetic, and women should undergo a complete medical examination including a wide variety of laboratory tests. (We touch on these tests in this chapter in the section "Medical causes of female hair loss" and in detail in Chapter 5.)

Genetic hair loss in women

In women, there's a distinct relationship between mother, sisters, aunts, and grandmothers when it comes to thinning hair patterns. When we take a careful history from women with thinning hair, far more than half of the women we interview with balding or thinning have female relatives with a similar problem. When one recognizes this in the family history, we generally ask these women to inquire on the course of the family balding patterns from a timeline perspective.

Genetic hair loss is relatively uncommon in women and is generally referred to as *female pattern hair loss* or *female androgenetic alopecia.* In women with this condition, the common pattern differs than that of men. Whereas the pattern in men follows the Norwood classification (refer to the earlier section, "Norwood classifications for measuring male pattern thinning"), the postmenopausal pattern in women is characterized by diffuse thinning starting just behind a normal hairline and extending to and beyond the swirl.

Unlike men, adult women with typical female postmenopausal androgenetic alopecia often have significant levels of miniaturization (decreased hair shaft thickness in some hairs and loss of hairs within the follicular unit) in the back and side of the scalp.

Miniaturization causes hair shafts to become thinner over time before falling out, and the higher degree of miniaturization present indicates an unstable hair loss process throughout the scalp.

In some women, the genetic pattern of hair loss is associated with an increase in male sex hormones (androsterone, testosterone, and DHT), but in most cases of genetic hair loss, it occurs when the sex hormone levels are normal.

Compared to men, the mechanism of balding in women is less well understood because their hair loss isn't as directly related to the presence of DHT. The enzyme aromatase appears to have a role in causing female hair loss and may partially explain the different pattern when compared to men. The loss of estrogens in postmenopausal women means that the protection against female genetic alopecia is withdrawn, bringing on the thinning.

Women who develop pattern balding later in life also have a genetic component to their hair loss, but the association is less strong. The changes in hormones that occur around menopause are an obvious contributing factor.

Because genetic hair loss presents itself differently in women than in men, a different classification system is used. Doctors use the Ludwig classification to describe the thinning that women experience. A Ludwig type I is associated with a mild widening of the part width. Patients who fall into type II have increased thinning with moderate widening of the part. Type III patients have significant widening of the part width. Figure 4-3 depicts types I through III.

A minority of women develop pattern balding in a distribution that's similar to men. These patients are better classified using the Norwood classification system. Because these women have hair loss mainly limited to the front and top of the scalp that doesn't affect the back and sides, they may be candidates for hair transplant surgery, which we discuss in Chapter 13. About 15 percent of women have this patterned balding.

Medical causes of female hair loss

Apart from genetics, female hair loss can stem from a variety of medical causes. This section looks at those causes, from the general to the more specific, including postpartum and menopausal hair loss.

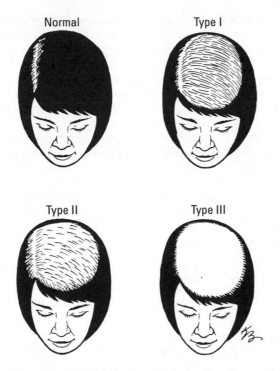

Figure 4-3: The Ludwig classification system for genetic hair loss in women.

Underlying medical conditions

In women, many medical conditions may cause hair loss, including the following:

- Thyroid disease
- Anemia
- Iron deficiency
- Weight loss induced by severe dieting or eating disorders
- Medication use (particularly oral contraceptives, beta-blockers, vitamin A, thyroid drugs, tranquilizers and sedatives, Coumadin, and prednisone)
- A variety of autoimmune diseases

See Chapter 5 for a full discussion of medical problems that cause hair loss.

As a woman experiencing hair loss, you should first be evaluated by a dermatologist to make sure that no underlying skin conditions are contributing to the hair loss. They may require a treatment different and may require a biopsy to rule out the presence of certain skin diseases like diffuse alopecia areata. Your family doctor can do the required blood tests for the various diseases that may be present. Dermatologists are the best to hone in on a diagnosis.

Blood tests check the following common contributors to female hair loss and can help rule out some identifiable medical conditions:

- **ANA (antinuclear antibody):** Used to test for lupus or other autoimmune diseases. This test is either positive or negative and further testing may be required if the initial screening tests are positive.

- **Iron:** Levels serum iron, TIBC (total iron binding capacity), and ferritin deficiencies in iron.

- **Estradiol:** This sex hormone indicates the status of ovarian output.

- **FSH (follicle-stimulating hormone):** This sex hormone indicates the status of ovarian output. This hormone reflects the status of a woman's ability to ovulate.

- **LH (luteinizing hormone):** This is a sex hormone indicates the status of ovarian outputa woman may be in her overall aging process. When she ovulates, this hormone stimulates the production of eggs.

- **Free testosterone:** May help the doctor understand a woman's ability to convert testosterone into estrogen. Most testosterone is bound to proteins in the blood and the free testosterone is easily converted into estrogen.

- **SHBG (sex hormone binding globulin):** Level indicates the status of male hormones.

- **TSH (thyroid-stimulating hormone):** Level indicates the presence of hyperthyroidism or hypothyroidism.

- **Total testosterone:** Largely bound to proteins in the blood.

It's important to note that even after a medical condition has been corrected, your hair loss may still persist perhaps because of a "switch" in your genetic makeup that's turned on when the medical insult occurs. After the hair loss starts, it may be difficult to turn off this switch. The hope is that your hair loss will slow down after your medical condition is treated or cured and any deficiency of your overall hormone balance is corrected.

Baby blues: Postpartum hair loss

Pregnancy alters a woman's overall hormone configuration in many different ways. When hormones change, hair becomes a target organ for change in some (but not all) women because the rapid growth of the hair cells reflects changes in the overall hormonal environment in the woman's body.

When you're pregnant, your production of the sex hormone estrogen increases, which prolongs the growth (anagen) phase of the hair cycle. During pregnancy, many women are delighted to discover that their hair is thicker and more lush. After the baby is born, however, estrogen levels drop and more hair lapses into the resting (telogen) phase. Consequently, your growing hair may fall out, and because the resting cycle lasts two to six months, it may take time to see the hair return to its growth phase.

Because hair grows at about ½ inch per month and doesn't start growing again until the rest cycle is complete, it can take up to a year for you to get your "old" hair back. In that period, you may think you're going bald; don't worry, you aren't. In nursing moms, the resting period can take longer than a year, and it may take more than a year for hair growth to return to previous levels.

Anemia and hypothyroidism also can contribute to postpartum hair loss. You can find out more about these medical conditions and others in Chapter 9.

Menopause-related hair loss

Over 50 percent of women going through the hormone fluctuations associated with menopause experience significant hair loss. The drop in estrogen levels in postmenopausal women may put the hair in a prolonged resting phase; this phase is particularly important for those women who have inherited female genetic hair loss. Unfortunately, doctors don't really understand the mechanisms by which the withdrawal of estrogen causes hair loss in women, but they know that it occurs. Women who lose estrogen support have many changes in their bodies, of which hair is only one. There are books written on the use of hormone supplements for managing menopausal changes in the body, and this book is not meant to deal with these complex issues.

Chapter 5

Diseases that Cause Hair Loss

· ·

In This Chapter

▶ Differentiating between scarring and non-scarring scalp diseases

▶ Understanding how lupus can affect hair

▶ Knowing what medications can cause hair loss

▶ Exploring other causes of hair loss

· ·

*A*lthough the most common cause of hair loss in adults is pattern thinning, it's not the only cause. A number of medical conditions can cause *alopecia,* the medical term for hair loss. Alopecia can occur as a disease in which hair loss is the predominant feature, or it may be a side effect from a disease or treatment of disease, such as alopecia caused by chemotherapy drugs.

Alopecia breaks down into two main categories, non-scarring and scarring. If properly treated, a *non-scarring* disorder can subside and hair can potentially grow back. With a *scarring* hair loss disorder, the hair follicles are permanently damaged; the chances of hair regrowth after the disorder is treated are very slight.

This chapter looks at the common medical causes of alopecia and their causes, courses, and cures.

 Visit the following Web sites to see photos of the various disorders discussed in this chapter:

http://dermatlas.med.jhmi.edu/derm/cd_lists.cfm

www.dermnet.com/moduleSearch.cfm

Without a Trace: Non-scarring Alopecia

Non-scarring hair loss disorders are generally reversible, but that doesn't mean that you shouldn't take them seriously. Here, we describe some of the most common causes of non-scarring hair loss, their symptoms, and their treatments.

Seeing circular bald spots: Alopecia areata

As if there aren't already enough difficult-to-pronounce terms in this book, here's another one: *alopecia areata.* Also called AA, alopecia areata is an autoimmune disease that causes hair loss (see the sidebar "What's an autoimmune disease?"). AA is sometimes called *spot baldness* because it causes round spots of hair loss. The disease, which is relatively common, tends to run in families and affects about 1 to 2 percent of the population in the United States. In about 2 percent of patients, the disease changes into a more diffuse form of hair loss, covering wider areas of the scalp.

Alopecia areata occurs when a person's white blood cells attack and destroy the body's hair follicles. After hair follicles are attacked, they stop producing hair, causing the distinctive localized bald patches that are the mark of alopecia areata. The hair loss usually occurs over a short period of time.

Severe alopecia areata can take two forms:

- ✔ **Alopecia totalis:** All hair on the scalp is lost.
- ✔ **Alopecia universalis:** All hair on the scalp is lost, along with hair on the eyebrows, eyelashes, and all other parts of the body.

Less severe alopecia areata can take these forms:

- ✔ **Alopecia areata monolocularis:** Baldness occurs in only one place on the scalp.
- ✔ **Alopecia areata barbae:** Hair loss occurs in patches in a man's beard.

AA can occur at any age, with most patients diagnosed between the ages of 15 and 29 and nearly half being under age 20. An equal number of men and women develop AA, and the disease occurs equally in every race.

Diagnosing the disorder

Alopecia areata doesn't follow a predictable path. Some patients feel burning or itching in the area of balding, but others don't. Eighty percent of patients have only one bald spot. The bald patches can be round or oval in shape, and expose smooth, bald skin.

The disease normally affects only the scalp, but other body hair also can be affected and aid in diagnosing the condition. Interestingly, if you have fingernail abnormalities such as small pits on the nail plate, you may also have alopecia areata. Atopic dermatitis (an allergic skin condition) and vitiligo, a disease that causes white patches on the skin, are also more common in people with AA.

An important diagnostic clue to alopecia areata is the presence of "exclamation point hairs" on the perimeter of the bald patch. These hairs form as the body attacks the lower portion of the hair follicle, and the damage produces a finely tapered end. As the hair continues to grow, it looks like a tiny spear stuck in the scalp. Eventually this hair will be lost, but its presence is a sign of alopecia areata in its active stage.

Your doctor may gently pull hair along the edge of a bald patch to determine whether you have alopecia areata. Healthy hair doesn't come out when pulled gently, but hair afflicted with alopecia areata is easily removed.

Exploring treatment options

If you're diagnosed with alopecia areata, the good news is that in 90 percent of cases, hair grows back on its own and no treatment is needed. The chances of regrowth are best when the condition is localized to just a few places on the scalp and the patient is over age 40. In younger patients, unfortunately, the condition tends to be more severe. If the disease progresses to alopecia totalis or alopecia universalis (refer to the earlier section, "Seeing circular bald spots: Alopecia areata"), no surefire treatment is available.

Options for treatment include:

✔ **Steroids:** One of the main functions of steroids is to reduce inflammation, but in patients with AA, steroids are used to stop the body's immune cells from destroying hair follicles. Your doctor may inject steroids directly into your bald patches or may prescribe a topical steroid cream that you can apply to the bald patches at home.

When the disease is too extensive to treat with multiple injections or topical creams, oral steroids are an option. Usually, you only take them for a short period of time because of the many side effects of long-term use, including osteoporosis, very fragile skin, and diabetes.

✔ **Minoxidil:** This medicine works because hair growth is a side effect of the drug that may directly affect bald spots. You apply it directly to the bald patches. Minoxidil is commonly used to treat pattern baldness, but for unknown reasons it also sometimes helps patients with AA.

✔ **Cyclosporine:** This potent immunosuppressant specifically inhibits T cells, the immune system cells that attack hair follicles in AA. Cyclosporine is most often given orally. It's more commonly used to treat other conditions such as psoriasis, and many physicians are hesitant to use it medicine to treat AA because it can cause kidney damage, high blood pressure, and suppress your body's immune system.

✔ **DNCB:** This chemical (full name *dinitrochioro benzene*) rapidly produces skin sensitivity. In some people with severe alopecia areata, continued application of DNCB (enough to produce a continuing rash caused by the activation of white blood cells to boost the local immune function). This caused hair regrowth in some individuals. It doesn't always work, however. You should take DNCB only under the strict supervision of a doctor who's experienced with this treatment.

What's an autoimmune disease?

Three diseases that can cause hair loss — alopecia areata, scleroderma, and lupus — are *autoimmune diseases.* But what is an autoimmune disease?

Your body's immune system serves to protect it from outside invaders, such as harmful bacteria and viruses. With an autoimmune disease, your immune system turns on itself and starts attacking components of your body. In other words, your body mistakenly thinks that some of its own cells are foreign, disease-causing cells, and so it attacks and tries to kill or damage those cells. Autoimmune diseases result from a failure of the immune system to distinguish between which cells belong in your body and which cells don't belong.

The cause of autoimmune diseases remains a mystery. They may have a genetic component because they tend to run in families. They're also much more common in women than in men, but doctors and researchers continue to hunt for the exact cause.

Hair today, gone tomorrow: Telogen effluvium

Telogen effluvium is a type of non-scarring hair loss characterized by sudden, widespread hair shedding. Normally, people lose 100 to 150 hairs each day, but you can lose more than 400 or more hairs daily with telogen effluvium! This disease can occur at any age and may be more common in women because of hormonal changes in menopause. It occurs equally in different races.

Telogen effluvium occurs when a large number of hair follicles suddenly decide to take a rest at the same time (the telogen phase; see Chapter 2 for more on the hair cycle). Then, three to four months later, this formerly resting hair sheds as new hair begins to take its place.

Why does a large portion of hair suddenly enter the resting phase and bring about an attack of telogen effluvium? Usually a traumatic event causes the condition (see the following list for some examples). Essentially, in times of stress, the body diverts its energies to something other than growing hair. As a result, the hair goes into a resting stage until the traumatic event subsides. The problem is that after the trauma, the hair can't just start growing again. It first has to be shed, and then you have to wait for new hair to grow in.

Common causes of telogen effluvium include the following:

✔ An acute illness accompanied by high fever

✔ A chronic illness, such as cancer

✔ Hormonal changes brought about by childbirth or stopping birth control

✔ Sudden changes in diet, including the conditions anorexia and bulimia

✔ Medications, such as those used to treat high blood pressure, cholesterol, and seizures

✔ Major surgery and general anesthesia

✔ Big life changes such as a divorce, death in the family, or loss of a job

People with telogen effluvium often seek help from a physician because the shedding is so sudden. Doctors often diagnose telogen effluvium with a hair pull test; pulling out significantly more than 10 percent of the hair indicates telogen effluvium in its early stage. The condition can be either *acute,* lasting less than six months, or *chronic,* lasting longer than six months. But there's some good news for telogen effluvium sufferers: After the hairs fall out, they start growing again, so hair loss from telogen effluvium usually isn't permanent. Be patient and your hair will grow back.

The fungus among us: Tinea capitis

By far the most common reason for hair loss in children is a fungal infection of the scalp called *tinea capitis*. This condition is rarely seen in adults. Depending on the severity of the infection, it can appear as a mild case of dandruff; reddened, circular areas of complete hair loss on the scalp that show whitish, scaly flakes; or a massive blister that covers the whole scalp. Often the infection is accompanied by swollen lymph nodes under the ear and on the back of the neck.

Outbreaks of tinea capitis aren't uncommon in schools. Doctors can make a definitive diagnosis by taking a fungal culture of the hair or looking at the hair under a microscope and noting the tiny fungal branches. The infection is treated with oral antifungal medicine usually taken for a period of several months.

When the infection is mild and treated early, any lost hair is expected to regrow. When the condition is associated with a lot of inflammation, scarred patches may form that are permanently devoid of hair. In this case, the condition should be viewed as a type of scarring alopecia (see the later section, "Scarring Conditions That Cause Hair Loss").

Thyroid conditions and hair loss

The *thyroid* is a small gland that resides on the front of your neck. It controls how your body makes proteins and burns energy; it also regulates your metabolism through production of thyroid hormone. Diseases of the thyroid gland can affect hair growth, which fortunately is non-scarring.

Diseases of the thyroid gland

When the thyroid gland produces either too much or too little thyroid hormone, it can have negative consequences for your hair. Fortunately, the following thyroid gland diseases can be detected with a simple blood test:

✔ **Hyperthyroidism:** When the body produces too much thyroid hormone, you may develop *hyperthyroidism*. Symptoms of hyperthyroidism include a rapid heartbeat, weight loss, heat intolerance, and nervousness. In addition, your hair becomes extremely thin and sparse.

✔ **Hypothyroidism:** When the body produces too little thyroid hormone, you may develop *hypothyroidism.* Symptoms of hypothyroidism include fatigue, cold intolerance, lack of energy, puffiness of the face, and dry skin. In addition, your hair becomes dry, brittle, coarse, and sparse.

The most common cause of hyperthyroidism in the U.S. is Grave's disease, an autoimmune disease (see the earlier sidebar "What's an autoimmune disease?"). The most common cause of hypothyroidism in the U.S. is Hashimoto's thyroiditis, also an autoimmune disease. In developing countries, lack of iodine in the diet is the most common cause of hypothyroidism. However, this cause is rare in the United States because iodine is added to table salt.

How thyroid conditions affect hair growth

Doctors aren't sure why patients with thyroid disease lose their hair. It could be because the thyroid hormone affects the body's metabolism, including the hair follicles, and so problems with the hormone cause hair regrowth to slow and hair to become thinner and possibly more brittle. This may result in loss of hair bulk. And if the hair shaft hasn't fully developed, the ends of the hair may split.

Whether or not the thyroid hormone has a direct effect on the condition of hair and its growth, acute thyroid disease is very stressful. As we explain in the section, "Hair today, gone tomorrow: Telogen effluvium," earlier in this chapter, stress can be an important factor in developing telogen effluvium, in which hair rapidly falls out after prematurely entering the resting phase of the hair growth cycle.

Medications given to treat thyroid dysfunction also can cause hair loss. For example, hair loss is a potential side effect of propylthiouracil, the most common medicine used to treat hyperthyroidism. Synthroid (levothyroxine), the most common drug used to replace thyroid hormone, also may cause hair loss. It's not known why these medications cause hair loss, but it's important for patients to be aware of their potential side effects.

Living with a thyroid condition and hair loss

If you suffer from thyroid disease and experience hair loss, you should see two important specialists: the endocrinologist, who can diagnosis and treat your thyroid condition; and the dermatologist, who can figure out the exact cause of your hair loss and determine if it's related to a thyroid disease. Hair loss can accompany many different conditions, so it's important to eliminate all other possible causes before assuming that a condition is thyroid related.

If your doctor determines that your hair loss is caused by thyroid dysfunction, be patient with treatment. Proper medical treatment and allowing time for your body to adjust to the new medication increase the likelihood that your hair will regrow. But you may have to wait out an entire hair cycle for this to occur, so it may take up to three years for your hair to return to normal.

Thyroid disease treatments

Patients with hypothyroid conditions (too little thyroid hormone in your body) are usually prescribed a drug called *synthroid*, which is essentially a replacement of the thyroid hormone. Hypothyroidism can be treated with any of the following:

- ✔ Medical therapy in combination with antithyroid drugs. When a person has too much thyroid hormone (hyperthyroid) they are often prescribed medicine that damages the thyroid gland so that it produces less thyroid hormone. At times, this treatment is overdone, so a person who was hyperthyroid becomes hypothyroid so that they need more thyroid hormone to bring the thyroid hormone to normal levels.

- ✔ The destruction of the thyroid gland in combination with radioactive iodine.

- ✔ Surgery to remove the thyroid.

If these treatments don't work, your doctor should consider treatments for simultaneously occurring androgenetic alopecia, or ANA (male pattern baldness that has a genetic cause; see Chapter 4 for more information). Thyroid disease may bring out the genetic defects of inherited balding so medicines used to treat ANA include topical minoxidil, spironolactone, and oral Finesteride (males only). Often there's no single reason for hair loss, and these medicines may help decrease hair loss when used with thyroid replacement therapy.

After you're diagnosed with thyroid disease and begin treatment, you may find that your hair loss begins to improve. However, if you continue to lose hair several months after your thyroid hormone levels have returned to normal, see your doctor to be sure another medical condition isn't causing your hair loss.

Other diseases that can cause hair loss

Almost any serious illness can cause temporary hair loss. Some of the most common are:

✔ **Anemia:** The most common type of anemia is due to iron deficiency. Decreased iron intake (seen in strictly vegetarian diets) or increased blood loss (sometimes associated with prolonged periods of heavy menstruation) may cause a drop in your iron level.

✔ **Diabetes:** Endocrine imbalances, stress, and poor circulation all can lead to hair loss in diabetic patients.

✔ **Malnutrition, including anorexia and bulimia:** These disorders produce hair loss particularly if there's a deficiency in zinc or essential fatty acids.

✔ **Psoriasis:** Treatments used for psoriasis or over-vigorous removal of plaques from the scalp can cause scalp inflammation, which may lead to hair loss. When this occurs, it is almost always from a person 'picking' at their hair plaques pulling out hair to produce traction alopecia.

All forms of chronic illness cause a metabolic shift of nutrients to the hair follicles and may bring on telogen effluvium (acute or chronic; refer to the earlier section "Hair today, gone tomorrow: Telogen effluvium" for an explanation). Telogen effluvium may last until the primary disease is resolved.

Accidents cause stress and can precipitate hair loss. In men with known genetic hair loss, stressful events can accelerate the process, which may not be reversible even after recovery. In women, hair loss can occur in a similar manner to acute telogen effluvium and reverses after full recovery from the accident.

A Potentially Permanent Change: Scarring Alopecia

Despite the sound of the name, scarring alopecia, also called *cicatricial alopecia,* doesn't always cause visible scars on top of your head; the scarring is usually beneath the scalp, where hair follicles are replaced with scar tissue. If severe, it can cause the surface of the scalp to appear smooth and shiny.

All scarring alopecias have similar microscopic features and show the body's immune cells attacking the skin and hair follicles. The changes in what we see can be quite similar with the changes of the non-scarring alopecias. Doctors categorize these conditions based upon the following:

✔ **Characteristics of the skin:** The skin loses its shine and texture and becomes dull and hard to the touch. The skin may erupt.

✔ **How hair reacts to the disease:** Most of these conditions exist in particular areas of the scalp and surrounding skin can be completely normal.

✔ **The presence of what may appear to be an infective component to the presentation:** It is not unusual for the skin to develop blister type changes with redness that appears infective.

✔ **How the disease starts and evolves over time:** The various scarring alopecias have distinct evolutionary changes in the skin over time and there may be other elements of the disease impacting other parts of the body. This is where the skill of the dermatologist plays an important role.

✔ **Family history of similar diseases:** Family history of the disease is common in alopecia areata.

✔ **The presence of weeping at the skin level may produce wetness:** Some of these diseases can also be dry and crusty, some have a normal skin, while others have a very fine thin skin over the involved areas.

Scarring alopecia occurs when the hair follicles are destroyed. If the condition attacks the hair follicles directly, it's called *primary cicatricial alopecia;* one example is lichen planopilaris (see the following bullets). Indirect follicle damage is called *secondary scarring alopecia;* examples include damage from radiation therapy or a burn injury to the scalp.

Relatively uncommon conditions that can cause permanent, scarring hair loss include:

✔ **Lichen planopilaris:** It often appears in the form of purplish bumps or red-to-purple rims around the hair follicles and can be on the scalp alone or associated with the skin condition lichen planus. Although the cause is unknown, it appears that the body's white blood cells attack the hair follicles and cause permanent damage to them.

✔ **Frontal fibrosing alopecia:** More common in postmenopausal women, this condition is characterized by large spaces that appear between hair follicles of normal diameter. A scalp biopsy will reveal many immune cells in the process of destroying the hair follicles they surround.

✔ **Pseudopelade:** This form of scarring alopecia looks like alopecia areata in its general shape. It's not a specific disease but rather a pattern of old or burned-out scarring alopecia, resulting from a variety of causes.

✔ **Dissecting cellulitis of the scalp:** This condition is characterized by multiple pustules and large cystic nodules in the scalp and can be associated with severe facial acne. It most commonly occurs at the back of the scalp. It's much more common in people of African descent.

A scalp biopsy can readily determine if hair loss is non-scarring or scarring and therefore permanent. However, determining exactly which scarring condition caused the hair loss can be difficult.

It's worth repeating that if you're experiencing hair loss, it's important to see your doctor to determine the type of loss and whether it's treatable. And if it is treatable, you should start your treatment as soon as possible in an effort to prevent permanent hair loss.

Lupus: A Scarring and Non-scarring Disease

Lupus is an autoimmune disease that causes inflammation of organ tissue (see the sidebar, "What's an autoimmune disease?," earlier in this chapter). Up to half of people with lupus experience hair loss at some point during the course of the disease; hair loss can occur in areas near the temples or be patchy and diffuse. The two main types of lupus are

✔ **SLE** (systemic lupus erythematosus), which is systemic (meaning it impacts many parts of the body) and may cause non-scarring hair loss. Although it's an autoimmune disease, SLE spares the hair follicles, so hair grows back after the disease is successfully treated.

✔ **DLE** (discoid lupus erythematosus), which is localized and may cause scarring hair loss. DLE causes irregular patches of hyperpigmented (skin that is dark) and hypopigmented (skin that appears almost white) skin, along with redness, scales, scarring, and hair follicles devoid of hair. The condition can occur anywhere on the body but is most common on the head and neck, particularly the scalp and ears.

General symptoms of lupus include reddish facial rashes, sensitivity to the sun, mouth ulcers, arthritis, which can be quite disabling, low-grade fevers, and persistent fatigue. Lupus most commonly affects women in the 20–50 age bracket. Blood tests diagnose the condition.

Systemic lupus is a serious disease, and most people who have it are concerned less with hair loss and more with the graver symptoms (such as severe arthritis, diseases of the kidneys and lungs). There's no specific treatment for hair loss associated with SLE, but medications used to treat the disease may also help with hair loss.

To complicate matters, some medications (such as Plaquenil) used to treat lupus can have the side effect of hair loss. If you recently started on a new medication to treat lupus and have noticed new onset hair loss, be sure to consult your doctor to see if the drug is causing your hair loss.

DLE is a much less serious condition than SLE. Oral medications such as Plaquenil and the local injection of steroids in the plaques of the scalp can control the disease, and if your doctor catches it early, localized hair loss caused by the plaques of DLE may be prevented.

May Cause Side Effects: Medications and Hair Loss

Some medications can do more than cure what ails you: They can cause you to lose hair. The list of drugs that may cause hair loss is huge, but here are a few of the more common ones:

- Acne medications, such as isotretinoin (Accutane)
- Antiinflammatory drugs, such as naproxen (Naprox), indomethacine (Indocin), and naproxen (Naprosyn)
- Antidepressives, such as paroxetine (Paxil), fluoxetine hydrochloride (Prozac), and sertraline hydrochloride (Zoloft)
- Beta blockers, such as nadolol (Corgard), propanolol (Inderal), metoprolol (Lopressor), and atenolol (Tenormin)
- Birth control pills
- Blood thinners, such as warfarin sodium (Coumadin) and heparin
- Cholesterol-lowering drugs, such as gemfibrozil (Lopid)
- Gout medications, such as allopurinol (Lopurin or Zyloprim)
- Seizure medications, such as trimethadione (Tridone)
- Ulcer medications, such as famotidine (Pepcid), cimetidine (Tagamet), and ranitidine (Zantac)

Other Causes of Hair Loss

Sometimes the disease process that results in hair loss actually has nothing to do with hair. For example, constant or deliberate hair pulling can result in loss of perfectly normal hair, and constant traction on hair from rubber bands or other hair accessories can cause perfectly normal hair to break off. This section looks at a two unique causes of hair loss.

Tearing your hair out: Obsessive compulsive disorders

The expression "I'm pulling my hair out" means the speaker is frustrated or perturbed. Everyone gets the urge to pull out their hair now and then, but for some people, literal hair pulling amounts to an obsessive-compulsive disorder.

An *obsessive-compulsive disorder* (OCD) is a psychiatric disorder in which a person tries to defuse his or her obsessive thoughts by repeatedly performing compulsive tasks. If you repeatedly tug at your hair, you have a type of OCD called *trichotillomania* (it's also known as "trich" or TTM). TTM is non-scarring, so your hair can grow back if you stop pulling and tugging. Usually people with trichotillomania pull scalp hair, but they may also yank hair from their eyebrows, eyelashes, and bodies.

The demographics of TTM

Trichotillomania sufferers fall into two groups:

- Those who intentionally pull out their hair because of an itch or feeling of pain. Sometimes they get a sense of pleasure from hair pulling.
- Those who pull out their hair by habit and may not realize they're doing it.

TTM is more common in children than adults, often striking in early adolescence. More women than men suffer from the disorder.

Often the dermatologist is the first to diagnose the problem and then sends the patient to a psychiatrist for treatment. Quite often, patients seek help for their hair loss without realizing that it's self-induced and that they have trichotillomania.

Treating TTM

Several treatment options are available for trichotillomania. If the sufferer is a child, cutting the hair short so that it can't be pulled may change the child's behavior over time.

For older children and adults, self-monitoring can also be a cure. You record the time and situation of hair pulling and the number of hairs pulled in an effort to increase awareness of the behavior. You also may seek behavioral modification or psychotherapy with a mental health professional. Medication is another option; the most common drugs used are antidepressants in the serotonin re-uptake inhibitors class. In addition, Clomipramine, a tricyclic antidepressant, may alleviate symptoms.

Prolonged hair pulling: Traction alopecia

If you have *traction alopecia,* you lose hair gradually due to prolonged tension on the follicles. People who wear their hair in tight braids, ponytails, and pigtails are most prone to this problem. It also can result from using tight roller curlers or repeatedly pulling the hair when straightening it. Because of these activities, traction alopecia is more prevalent in women than men and much more commonly seen in people of African descent. If caught early, it's reversible, but persistent traction alopecia can lead to scarring.

The problem first appears as patchy areas of hair loss on the periphery of the scalp; eventually these areas can extend further into the scalp and result in large areas of hair loss. The treatment — not putting any more tension on the hair — seems simple, but getting patients to change old habits is never as easy as it seems.

It's essential to detect the condition early so it can be treated before large amounts of hair are permanently damaged. Late diagnosis often means irreversible loss, and no treatment can make the lost hair grow back again. The only way to restore the hair is through hair transplantation, which is only practical if not too much of the patient's hair has been lost. (Turn to Chapter 13 for more on hair transplantation.)

Enduring Hair Loss with Chemotherapy

Chemotherapy is the treatment of disease with powerful drugs meant to kill rapidly growing cancerous cells. Because the drugs are so potent, chemotherapy has many side effects, one of which is hair loss. Chemotherapy targets not just cancer cells but all rapidly growing cells, including hair follicle cells, which is why chemotherapy often causes severe hair loss.

Not all chemotherapy drugs cause hair loss; your doctor will tell you if the drug or drugs you're taking have this side effect. Some newer chemotherapy drugs are made to specifically target certain cells and spare your hair.

Still, if you're receiving chemotherapy, it's likely that all your hair in the actively growing phase will fall out. Because 90 percent of hair is in this phase of the hair growth cycle at any given time, essentially all your hair may fall out during treatment. Different drugs cause different hair loss patterns; with paclitaxel (Taxol), the loss is sudden, while cyclophosphamide (Cytoxin) causes hair to thin but not fall out altogether.

The good news is that your hair usually starts to grow back within six to eight weeks after you stop treatment. You may ask your doctor about topical minoxidil, which has been shown to accelerate the regrowth of hair by almost two months. When your hair does grow back, it may initially be curlier and have a different texture, but it should return to its old self within a year.

Part III
Creative Techniques for Concealing Hair Loss

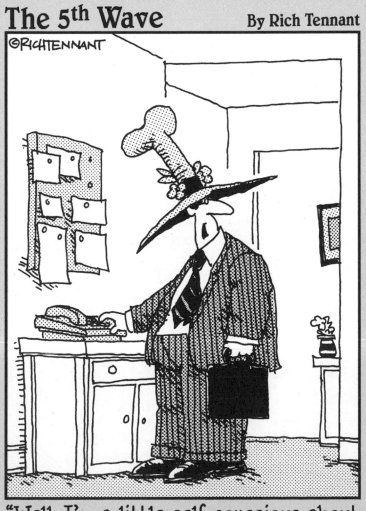

The 5th Wave   By Rich Tennant

"Well, I'm a little self-conscious about my hair loss, and I think wearing a toupee would make me look ridiculous."

In this part . . .

Ready for some sleight of hand? From covering balding or thinning hair with any of a variety of hair
replacement systems (think toupees, wigs, weaves, and
more) to taking a little bit of hair and make it appear to be
more than it is, concealing hair loss is easier than pulling a
rabbit out of a hat. This section provides detailed coverage of your coverage options.

Chapter 6

Toupee or not Toupee?

*T*he practice of using toupees and wigs to cover hair loss goes back to the beginning of recorded history, and the jokes about toupees blowing away and wigs going askew have been around almost as long. A *toupee* is a small piece of hair (real or synthetic) on a mesh or fabric foundation that's worn to cover a bald or thinning area of scalp. Wigs cover more area than toupees and are known by many interchangeable names — hairpieces, rugs, units, hair systems, systems, or just pieces. For simplicity, we refer to both wigs and toupees as *hair replacement systems,* both in this chapter and throughout the book.

People turn to hair replacement systems for many reasons. For some, hair restoration surgery isn't an option due to cost or other factors; other people need a wig just for a short time because of hair loss from chemotherapy or another health-related temporary hair loss situation (see Chapter 5 for disorders that cause temporary hair loss).

In this chapter, we introduce you to the different types of hair replacement systems, addressing both their pros and cons as well as the care and maintenance they require. We also talk about methods for attaching these systems and the best ways to keep your hair in place while you live an active lifestyle.

A Brief History of "Rugs"

The earliest known example of a hair system was found in a tomb near Hierakonpolis, an ancient city in Egypt. The tomb and its contents date to 3200–3100 BC. As necessity is the mother of invention, and to address the balding problem, the hair system more resembling what's available today was later invented in the form of toupees or wigs.

Powerful men throughout history were self conscious about balding. It's known that Julius Caesar, who felt that his bald head had to be addressed, was known to have tried wearing a hair system, and King Louis XIII began wearing wigs to camouflage his balding condition in the 17th century. Due to King Louis XIII's tremendous influence, wigs soon became the fashion throughout France.

In England, King Charles II was restored to the throne after his exile in Versailles, where he was exposed to the French wig craze. The English, not to be outdone by the French, followed the fashion. The use of hair systems grew in the United States in the 19th century as well.

By the 1950s, it's estimated that over 350,000 American men wore hair systems, out of a potential 15 million wearers. With only about one percent of the market captured, the opportunities for hair systems seemed limitless. Hair system manufacturers helped to build credibility for their products starting in 1954, when several wig makers advertised hair systems in major magazines and newspapers. This opened the wig market to the men who knew they had a problem but didn't know what to do about it.

With advertising came acceptance of hair systems, and improvements in craftsmanship, pioneered by Max Factor, advanced the wig-making art of the time. Since that time, some national organizations like Hair Club for Men, sprung up to offer hair systems to a wide variety of men through heavy television promotion. For those of you old enough to remember the famous line Sy Sperling uttered in his commercials: "I'm not only the Hair Club president, I'm also a client." This was one of the more successful ads that helped make this industry, and it quickly became a phenomenon.

The heavy promotion on television gave rise to a new industry where hair salons all over the world started to exploit the market for hair systems. Almost every city had some specialty shop selling hair systems, and as a result of the heavy promotion, the quality of the hair systems got better and better.

Today's Hair Replacement Systems

Today's hair systems are quite an improvement over the powdered wigs of the 1700s. Many are made from human hair, resulting in a more natural feel and appearance. This section weighs the advantages and disadvantages of hairpieces, explains the attachment systems available, and prepares you for the care and upkeep of your hair replacement system.

Weighing the pros and cons of hair systems

Hair systems were the only option for balding prior to the late 1950s, when doctors developed hair transplantation. Today, for men whose baldness is very extensive and who don't have enough hair for a hair transplant, a hair system may be the only alternative to simply shaving the scalp. The cost and the final appearance of a hair system varies with the materials used and the expertise of the maker. Cost for a system also varies based on the total costs for marketing and commission sales. Most clients have two hair systems so that they can wear one while the other is in the shop.

The major advantages of wearing a hair system are that

- The initial cost can be relatively low.
- You get a fast and easy result (within a few hours) without a surgical procedure.

Some major disadvantages to hair systems include:

- A rapid change in appearance when the hair system is first used
- Lack of durability
- Need for frequent cleaning and repairs
- Need for duplicates for when one is "under repair"
- Potentially unnatural frontal hairline
- Unpleasant smell from scalp sebum (natural oil) buildup
- Accelerated hair loss caused by the hair system

All hair systems are fragile and must be returned to the maker regularly for cleaning and upkeep; even with this attention, they usually last only a year or two. Sun, salt water, human sweat, chlorine in swimming pools, and harsh shampoos all shorten the life of a hair system.

The highest quality and most natural-looking hair systems are custom-made and may cost thousands of dollars. They're made of high-quality human hair carefully matched to the original hair of the client. The hairs, singly or in a few bundles, are skillfully tied around the threads of the foundation netting and knotted so that they may follow the pattern of natural hair growth or lie in a direction that maximizes layering. Hair layered from side to side tends to cover better and, like a thatched roof, blocks light from penetrating the wig (which is important because one doesn't want the hair system to be seen through). Good cover is important for the users and a secure fit is critical because the new wearer will be most concerned about the feel of the hair system on their head and their concern that the hair system might just fall off.

Considering manufacture, upkeep, and replacement, even the average hair system isn't cheap, and you must expect continued expense throughout your life as long as you wear a system.

The hairs of less expensive hair systems may be made of artificial fibers or animal hair; cheap hair systems made from artificial fibers are less durable and begin to look fuzzy very quickly, so you must replace them at frequent intervals. Human hair has the most natural appearance and behavior, and the most common and affordable hair systems are traditionally made from Asian hair that's dyed or bleached to approximate Caucasian coloring. Asian hairs are used because they're generally coarse, straight, and strong, making them easier to work with. The costs of hair supplies from salons in developing Asian countries was far lower than from traditional European sources. However, the texture may be so different from a person's natural hair that the final result doesn't look convincing. Also, although Asian hair is very strong, the bleaching and toning processes make it brittle and dry, making it vulnerable to breakage.

Keeping your hair from falling apart

Hair systems start with a section of netting called the *foundation*. The netting is cut and molded to approximate the size and shape of the bald scalp area in a custom-made hair system; it also can be more extensive in design, covering not only the bald area but also covering the existing hair around it to make the transition from hair system to normal hair more transparent.

Human hair is fragile and the oils, wax, and sebum that is meant to protect your living hair, becomes a liability for the hair system. The hair in a hairpiece can't replace itself as growing hair does and oils, wax, and sebum can't flow to the hair shaft because the foundation stands between your scalp and the artificial hair. With a lessened ability to clean the scalp from sebum and oil buildup, the hair systems accumulate this buildup. This means that you need to wash the hair system to get rid of the oil and sebum buildup or replace the hair system at intervals that depend upon the quality of the system and your requirements for keeping your hair looking perfect — or just good enough becomes a problem.

Synthetic hair fibers aren't as susceptible to injury unless you wash the hair system too frequently, heat them (or perm them) to a temperature that melts or chemically alters the fibers, or use products on the system that aren't easily removed.

Some people choose to style their hair system with perming equipment, rollers, hot irons, and hair dryers. This styling opens up the hair system to damage just as the same processes do on a normal head of hair (see Chapter 3 for more information on these processes in normal hair).

Setting up a cleaning schedule

Some types of hair systems are designed to be removed at night to allow you to wash your scalp and then reapply the hair system in the morning. When your scalp is cleared of the day's buildup of sebum and oils, the hair system will stay cleaner longer. Simple washing of the hair system doesn't remove skin cells, skin oils, shed hair, and other debris that accumulates in the foundation and in the hair fibers of your hair system. Either you learn to clean your own hair system on a regular basis or you bring it in for service and cleaning to keep it clean and odor free. A spare is an absolute necessity, possibly two. For those people who use hair systems that are made to stay on the head for weeks at a time, there is no real viable option for keeping down the odor and removing the oils and sebum that builds up every day. Cleaning/washing the hair system while it is still on your head is not a viable option for most people for two important reasons including:

1. The sebum and oils will stay below the foundation even if it is washed. Only the hair is really subject to washing.

2. The hair system that stays on your head after washing will remain wet for some time. Wearing a wet hair system is like

wearing your wet towel without giving it the opportunity to dry. We all know the musty odor of a wet cloth that is confined to a closed space.

Cleaning your hair system with it off your head will allow you to get to the foundation and remove the oils and sebum, but if you scrub it too vigorously, you can destroy the hair system relatively easily. There is clearly some balance between washing and preserving the integrity of the hair system. Drying it with a lukewarm hair dryer setting deals with that musty smell discussed earlier.

The attachment mechanism for the hair system is critical. It is always best to be able to get the hair system off so attachments with tape may work well for this purpose (see attachment mechanisms later in this chapter).

For most wearers, the initial expense of owning more than one hair system is justified by the increased lifespan of the hair systems because they can be switched while being washed.

Creating a natural-looking frontal hairline

It's not enough to just plop a toupee or wig — even a good one — on your head and forget about it. One of the problems with hair replacement systems is the appearance of the frontal hairline. Unless you have natural hair remaining in your frontal hairline, the foundation of the hair system may be highly visible, separating it visually from the scalp and leaving an artificial-looking hairline. Making this space appear normal is maybe the most challenging part of the manufacturer's job. Most hair systems utilize a style where the hair is actually combed forward over the hairline to hide it from direct observation. When there is bright light, the leading edge of almost all hair systems can be seen, so a forward combing styling may be critical to the disguise.

The best frontal meshes that extend from the hair system are customized to match your skin color and may be see through. The hair fibers at the hairline should be thinner than the hair used in the rest of the hair system. This is particularly important when the system uses coarse hair. As an alternative, the front hairs of the system can be cut short so that they fall forward, camouflaging the seam at the front edge of the hair system. Multiple hair thicknesses on the front of a hair system tend to increase the costs.

The time investment to manage the fine mesh is considerable and may be difficult for you to do yourself if you have anything but a completely bald front. If you still have natural hair growing at your hairline, shaving it for such attachments is ideal because any natural hair present (it grows at a rate of about ½ inch per month) causes significant problems in the ability to maintain the attachment beyond a week or so, but shaving the head and using tapes or glues will eventually cause traction alopecia and a loss of whatever hair you had there before you started wearing the hair system.

Many high-end hair system suppliers offer weekly services to reattach these hair systems and recreate the delicate frontal transition zone. The flipside is that this care makes the process more time-consuming than a monthly hair cut would be.

Attaching Your Hair

The greatest worry for anyone who wears a hair system is that it will unexpectedly come off in public. This fear can dictate your daily activities and keep you from doing things you like to do — you may avoid going outside on a windy or rainy day or pass on a day of water-skiing. But rest assured that manufacturers have put a great deal of effort into devising methods to attach hair systems securely. Each method has advantages and disadvantages, which is why this section helps you assess your options for keeping your hair where it belongs.

In general, the following methods are used for attaching a hair system.

- ✔ **Glue:** The area that the hair system covers is shaved or the hair is clipped very short, and you use glue around the outer edge of the hair system to hold it in place.

- ✔ **Clips:** You apply the clips attached to your hair system to the surrounding fringe of normal hair.

- ✔ **Double-sided tape:** The tape is attached to your hair system, and you stick it to your shaved scalp.

- ✔ **Weaves:** The weave is a different beast. It sews hair that you have into the foundation mesh. The hair anchors the hair system to your scalp, but the hair continues to grow so the hair system become looser over time (½ inch of growth per month can be expected). Most weaves need to be tightened every 7–10 days. Traction alopecia results from chronic use of weaves.

Loose glue changes a life

Joey loved baseball and played every weekend. At age 22, he got a hair system attached professionally with glue. When he was 26 years old and playing baseball every weekend, an accident on the field changed Joey's life. After hitting a double, Joey saw the pitcher hesitate and, seeing his opening, Joey ran for third base. He slid to the base but left his hair system some 10 feet behind him. It came off with his hat, exposing the front of his shaven bald head where the glue had been.

The crowd was in hysterics, and in the dugout, Joey's teammates were not kind about his hair loss. That was the last time Joey ever played baseball. He also lost contact with all his teammates who had such a good time at his expense. Loose glue changed the course of Joey's life.

Gluing it in place

A properly glued hair system is secure and comfortable for the wearer (some say it's the most comfortable attachment method available). You must redo the glue every 10 to 14 days because your scalp skin sheds under the hair system and eventually the system will loosen and come off. The opportunity to wash the hair system when it is re-glued is available to each user. Some people take enough command of their hair systems to wash them while others just use their spare while the hair system is being serviced and washed. During servicing, repairs on the hair system can also be made and these include: replacing hair that has come out, reattaching the hair to the foundation, and styling or color alterations to account for the exposure to the environment of the wearer.

Glued hair systems don't breathe easily (meaning they don't allow much air to circulate). Combine that with the fact that you remove it less often than other hair systems to clean both your head and the system, and you can understand why you should wash your hair system frequently enough to minimize any odor from the body's sweat and bacterial buildup underneath.

Every person who uses glue as an attachment mechanism develops a comfortable routine for removal and reattachment. Wearers often turn to those who sell and service the hair systems to handle this process.

Getting a professional to remove, reattach, and wash your glued hair system must be calculated into the total cost of the system.

Glues and clips are used frequently to attach weaves and wefts, two types of hair systems that we cover later in this chapter. When these systems are removed, normal hair may be pulled out because the bonding is often very secure and almost permanent. Great care should be taken not to put too much glue on the point of bonding the weave or weft to your natural hair. Some of the bonding mechanisms that glue the wefts to your scalp can last for as long as a few months, although this would be unusual.

Snapping and clipping

You may choose to attach your hair system with metal snaps or clips sewn to the foundation netting that fasten directly to your natural hair.

- ✔ **Metal snaps** are tied or sewn to the foundation and to your hair, which means they must be relocated as your natural hair grows out and the attachment loosens. Some of the advantages of clips and snaps are that

  - They're usually very secure once you get used to them.

  - The hairpiece is easily removed so you can cleanse your scalp and wash your hair as frequently as desired.

- ✔ **Metal clips** are ideal for affixing a hair system during the transition phase following a hair transplant when a client wants to cover his baldness while the new hair grows in.

One concern of clips is that the point of attachment to the existing hair may create localized balding from traction (called traction alopecia and explained in Chapter 5). Frequently relocating the clips to different areas of the hair system may postpone the appearance of traction alopecia, but sooner or later a bald area will develop at the point of attachment on the scalp.

Drilling it in: Don't try this at home!

One "clever" surgeon invented a snap system for attaching hair systems in which the snaps are anchored to the skull with drill-holes made in the bone. Bone cement was used to seal the snap, with the edge of one snap brought through the skin. The surgeon found some neurosurgical friend to affix the clips to his skull. He was promoting this technique, using his own head as an example. Could he have had a screw loose himself? We'll let you decide that for yourself.

Sticking it on with tape

Tape with adhesive on both sides is one of the simplest methods of attaching a hair system. It's particularly handy for removing the hair system at night to wash your scalp thoroughly. This attachment method generally requires that the scalp is shaved under the taped section.

In spite of its good points, double-sided tape does have some disadvantages, including the following:

✔ Tape can leave a sticky residue of adhesive on the skin and on the net foundation of your hair system.

✔ The tape often takes dead skin cells with it when you remove the hair system from your scalp. These skin flakes eventually build up on the tape, and as the skin flakes decay, they develop a pungent odor.

✔ With the skin buildup on the tape, the tape becomes less effective and must be changed and replaced.

✔ Tape tends to become unstuck when the hair system is pulled or when you sweat. For this reason, this type of attachment is especially unsuitable if you like to exercise or spend time in hot, humid, sunny climates.

✔ The stickiness of tape is vulnerable to swimming and diving, activities that tend to loosen the attachment of taped hairpieces.

Tips for keeping your hair tied down

As we mention earlier in this chapter, when you wear a hair system of any kind, one of your biggest concerns — and perhaps the root of your self-consciousness — is keeping it in place. No one wants to find themselves in the embarrassing situation of dealing with fly-away hair.

All attachment methods can be vulnerable under certain circumstances (which we address in the earlier sections on each method), but there are things you can do to ensure a tight connection between your scalp and your hair system. Here are a few ideas:

✔ **Change the glue or tape frequently.** The fresher the glue or tape, the more secure the bond will be.

✔ **If you use clips, also use glue or tape.** Combinations of attachment mechanisms add to attachment security.

✔ **Keep an open mind and experiment with the alternative attachment methods if you're not happy with the one you usually use.**

Attaching extensions: Weaves and wefts

If you have hair to work with, you can enhance it by using hair extensions in the form of weaves or wefts. Hair extensions come in various sizes and lengths and are groupings of synthetic or natural hair that are placed into your hair to add bulk to it.

Change isn't always a good thing

Michael wore his hair system to work, taking it off after work and at some social activities around the house. His hair system stylist, Sylvia, called one day to report a new advance in the product line — a lace front — that would help make Michael's hair system less detectable. That was a sticking point for Michael, so he headed to the hair system office. Sylvia recommended that Michael get the new lace front, which was a very fine nylon mesh with softer hair than the front of his existing hair system, which was made of a harsh, coarse hair and without transparent mesh. He enthusiastically agreed to give it a try.

Michael's method of attachment was clips attached to the sides and back of his hair system, and he had a considerable amount of thin hair at his frontal hairline. When Sylvia offered to shave the front of his hairline in order to glue on the new lace front, Michael refused the shave, saying that he didn't want to take such a drastic step until he was sure he liked it. So Sylvia glued the lace mesh in place, over Michael's normal hair in front.

When Michael got home, he felt uncomfortable as the glue pulled on his forehead and his frontal hairs, so he decided to go back to his previous attachment, using the spare hair system he kept at home. Unfortunately, when he tried to take off the glued lace front, it would not come off. He panicked and immediately called Sylvia, but the office was closed. He didn't sleep that night because the hair system tugged on his frontal hair, and he couldn't remove it as he did every night with the clipped system. In the morning, Michael returned to the office and had Sylvia remove the lace front with acetone and alcohol, but the whole experiment pulled out most of the hair he had at his frontal hairline. The lesson of this story is that everything has its price, and your comfort level with whatever you choose, is critical to commanding your independence.

✔ **Synthetic hair extensions:** Hairs are be attached to each other by putting heat to one end and fusing the hairs together. The small groupings of 20 to 50 fibers (hairs) may be attached to the base of your own hair with heat fusion, adhesive, clamping, wax, or braids.

The use of synthetics reduces the cost of hair extensions because fibers of monofilament are less expensive than human hair.

✔ **Natural hair extensions:** Hairs are attached as groups of hair. They can be affixed to a foundation (a weft) or they can be affixed to each other. The extensions consisting of grouped hairs can also be glued to your hair. When these extensions are glued to your existing hair, your original hair can grow and the extensions will move further away from the scalp as your hair grows.

Weaving a system in place

People often refer to a *weave* as a hair system, but it's really more of an attachment method. A weave involves a hair system on a mesh foundation; strands of your natural hair are woven through the edges of the foundation to secure the weave. This woven attachment method holds the hair system to your scalp very securely and naturally because of its many points of attachment.

Weaves can be used for hair systems as a mechanism of attachment. They can also be used to braid groups of hairs or individual hairs to the person's own hair. In theory, a single hair woven or braided to a single hair may be best, but that may be impractical considering the shear number of braids needed.

Hair systems secured with weaves require adjustment as the hair grows in order to keep the system tight to your scalp. After two weeks, your natural hair will have grown out about ¼ inch, and the hair system will move easily as an entire unit when touched.

With braided weaves to groups of hair, your natural hair is put into horizontal cornrows. Braids placed well behind the frontal edge of your hair can add bulk without detection. Your own hair can be weaved with the new hair (synthetic or natural hair), or threads or human hair or artificial hair may be used to enhance the fullness. The greater the number of attachment point, the more secure will be the impact. The greater the numbers of braids, the thicker the hair will appear.

Weaving braids of hair to your own hair can produce traction hair loss particularly because this attachment approach is left on for longer periods of time (a few months in some people). They only become problems when the attached hair moves too far away from

the scalp as your natural hair grows out. With braids, it's also difficult to lubricate or wash your hair because it's caught up in the
braid. Hair that is braided is often more brittle.

Weaves almost always pull on existing hair, some of which already
may be weakened by the balding process. But even if the hair isn't
already weakened, the constant pulling of the weave eventually
produces traction alopecia at the points of attachment (this also
happens with wefts, which we explain in the next section). For this
reason, you should have weave attachment points relocated often
to different areas of the scalp.

With good relocation, wefts can add substantial bulk to your existing hair without causing any permanent damage to your natural
hair. Wefts can also be moved to different locations frequently.
Unfortunately, many technicians who apply these wefts don't
understand the importance of moving them, so it is incumbent on
the wearer to direct the process as the wefts are reattached.

You also have the option of weaving artificial hair with the real hair
without a mesh foundation. One company invented special clips to
attach strands of artificial or human hair to the bottom of the shaft
of growing hair (almost one for one). Attaching this hair system is
a tedious process requiring a very hefty fee (in the $50,000 range)
and expensive weekly adjustments to tighten the strands of hair
and move them back toward the scalp as the hair grows out. The
normal hair acts as the anchor that holds the attached hair as your
normal hair grows out. Many similar services have been developed
at different facilities for far less costs, but unfortunately, all these
techniques cause traction alopecia.

Using wefts

As mentioned earlier in this chapter, a *weft* is a type of hair system.
It's usually a linear strip of human or synthetic hair that's bonded
to a latex or fabric strip. Wefts tend to be longer than the systems
used in weaves (braids of hair to hair), and they generally contain
more than 50 hairs or synthetic hair fibers. They may require more
points of attachment. They also provide more hair bulk than
weaves.

Wefts that are made with human hair woven into mesh are more
expensive than those that are pressed together with a machine and
glued to the mesh foundation. Regardless, the wefts should match
your hair color and hair thickness. After they're applied, they're
cut down to the length that fits with your hair style.

The wefts can be woven into place using your natural hair, which is
passed through the mesh with appropriate sewing needles and
then knotted. Another attachment method involves the use of

adhesive glue that holds the weft onto the parted hair or scalp. This bond creates a barrier for fingers getting down to the scalp when someone tries to run their fingers through your hair.

Attaching wefts with adhesive is fast and less expensive than other attachment methods, although it does usually require a professional to do it well. Clips allow flexibility for the user who wishes to apply the weft on their own.

There's no telling how long wefts will stay in place. For some people, their wefts stay attached for many weeks. But for others, the wefts may loosen up with the first shampoo. Natural hair oils cause the bond to lose its adhesive properties if it is glued, and an edge of a weft may lift off of the attached hair. If you use glue attachments, in order to help your wefts stay in place as long as possible, we recommend that you comb the hair very carefully and avoid perming your hair unless you use a salon that has experience combining hair styling with the advantages of the weft.

Attachment no-nos

Three attachment techniques require special attention because of the risks and serious consequences involved: sew-ons, tunnels, and the implantation of artificial fibers. We mention these techniques only to warn you against them. The damage of a scarred scalp is very difficult to hide or cover, and all three of these techniques will permanently scar your scalp. In our practices, we see patients seriously deformed by these techniques and always advise against them.

Sewing it on

With sew-ons, the hair system is stitched directly onto your scalp with an encircling, permanent surgical suture. This procedure is illegal in the U.S. and most European countries. Unfortunately, in New Jersey, a few companies have been able to use this dangerous technique for years despite attempts by the New Jersey attorney general to block them. They sidestep the law by employing retired doctors with a valid medical license to sew them into the scalp. The hair systems are attached to the stitch that is placed through the skin of the scalp. If this turns you off, we include it to dissuade anyone from considering this barbaric technique.

Skin is a more complex organ than most people realize. One of the skin's essential functions is to prevent bacteria and viruses in the environment from entering the bloodstream and reaching the vital organs. A suture through the skin leaves a small hole that allows bacteria to migrate into the fatty tissue under the skin. Long-term sutures through the skin often result in infection and abscesses (tender masses full of pus and bacteria).

Many sutures incite enough of a reaction to cause the suture to be rejected and extruded by the skin, tearing a large hole in the scalp. (Most sutures in the scalp are rejected by the person's body.) Surgical sutures left in the skin for too long need to be replaced, which is part of the profit of the sew-on business. This process of expelling the sutures is hastened when any traction is applied.

Between the sutures, the scars that they cause, and the recurrent infections, a wall of scar tissue gradually builds up in a circle around the sutured wounds. This encircling scar may eventually cause blood supply problems to the central portion of the scalp, and a thin, parchment-like layer of scar tissue may replace the skin in the center of the scalp. Any permanent hair that was present in the area surrounded by the suture is killed off. The damage from this process is permanent and the pain from the complications of this approach can be unbearable.

Tunneling grafts into the scalp

With this technique, tunnels are created in the skin of your scalp. These tunnels are made from small skin flaps from your own scalp skin. To make them permanent, skin grafts are often taken from another area of the body. Usually you get three tunnels: one in the front and two in the back. Plastic or nylon hooks are sewn to your hair system, and the hooks are inserted into the tunnels. The attachment is quite secure, and you can easily remove and replace the hair system without a visit to a wigmaker's salon. The best part of these tunnel grafts is that once they are in and secure, they are completely painless.

The obvious disadvantage of this procedure is that it involves minor surgery, and you must ask yourself if the punishment fits the crime. The tunnel grafts create a deformity that looks like handles to a suitcase. If the tunnels are removed later, permanent scars remain in the scalp. With enough donor hair, hair transplants may cover the scars on the back of the head left by the tunnels; however, the scar in front may be more difficult to conceal. And if you may need a hair transplant in the future to cover the damage from tunnels, why not just have a hair transplant in the first place?

Planting artificial fibers

The manufacturer of a synthetic polymer claims that its products look and feel like human hair. The material comes in small bundles of fibers that are implanted directly into the scalp. It's most widely used in Japan and elsewhere in Asia but not in the U.S. or many European countries.

Be careful about considering this option, as its safety is in question. The artificial fibers can cause many problems, not the least of which is scalp infection, which can be severe and difficult for the body to fight off because the fibers are embedded into the skin (similar to the sew-on sutures; refer to the earlier section, "Sewing it on"). Thousands of artificial fibers go through the scalp, and an average of 15 to 25 percent of the fibers are pushed out of the scalp each year. Initially, the results are quite remarkable and almost bald men look like they have a crew cut, but the price that one pays becomes more evident over time as infections occur, and the fibers are expelled. Scarring remains after all of the artificial fibers are expelled by the body.

It's almost impossible to treat the infections from these artificial fibers without removing the foreign material. The artificial fibers are brittle and tend to break off at the skin level, leaving bits of foreign debris under the skin that festers, swells, and produces pockets of pus. Infection caused by fiber implants also may cause premature loss of natural hair follicles adjacent to the artificial fibers. Over time, inflammation may destroy the scalp to the extent that further hair transplants of any kind are difficult or impossible.

Aside from potential scalp infection, the artificial fibers have an unnatural, stiff texture that doesn't feel like real hair. Combing is difficult because traction can break the fibers or pull them out, and using a hair dryer on them causes the fibers to frizz. Damage to the fibers above the skin level is permanent.

With so many problems and the fact that the process is illegal in most countries, one wonders why companies that make artificial fiber implants are still in business. The answer is simply profits. Anyone in the U.S. who sells these systems should be immediately turned over to the state medical boards.

Women and Hair Systems

As we explain in Chapters 4 and 5, women suffer from genetic thinning more often than outright baldness. The exception is about 15 percent of women, who experience frontal balding, develop a pattern similar to the Norwood classifications Class IIIA or IVA pattern of balding seen in men. We discuss this classification system in Chapter 4. Essentially, this type of balding goes from front to back. When a woman has this pattern, she may or may not lose the frontal ⅓ inch of hair but the hair extending as far back as about 3 inches may become very bald or very thin.

Women frequently treat genetic hair thinning themselves using hair systems that clip onto existing hair, but other attachment methods are possible as is discussed earlier in this chapter. The use of attachments is often a styling decision intended to thicken finer hair, because the holy grail for women is thick, luxurious hair — the type heavily promoted in magazine and television ads to the tune of billions of dollars annually.

As a woman, your options for attaching a hair system to your natural hair are

- ✔ Clips that attach close to the scalp.

- ✔ Weaves (discussed in the section, "Weaving a system in place," earlier in this chapter), in which small hair systems are woven into your hair.

- ✔ Wefts (discussed in the section "Using wefts"), in which long strips of hair are glued into the base of your hair.

African American women in particular are prone to alopecia, the fancy, medical name for hair loss. The use of thermal or chemical hair straightening products and hair braiding or weaving are styling techniques that place African American women at higher risk for various forms of "traumatic" alopecia than their Caucasian counterparts.

For example, tight braids that have pulled back the hair since childhood cause a substantial amount of traction alopecia in African American women. And traction alopecia has pushed many African American women to wear full wigs because the hair on the sides (which is often lost from the traction alopecia) isn't easily hidden with even a small wig or any other hair replacement systems.

Adding Up the Costs of Hair Systems

The cost of a hair system is highly variable because it depends on so many factors. This section looks into the practical financial costs as well as those costs that you may not think of right away — psychological effects and the possible lasting effect on your natural hair.

Starting with financial costs

Dollars-wise, the cost of a hair system depends on a number of factors. And there's no one-time-only cost when it comes to hair replacement systems, especially because you may want to purchase up to three hair systems: one to wear, one as a spare, and one to wear if the others need repair.

Here are the basic variables that affect how much of a hit your bank account takes thanks to your hair systems:

- ✔ The quality and durability of the system
- ✔ The manufacturer's marketing costs
- ✔ Monthly maintenance costs for cleaning and repairing what hair has fallen out
- ✔ Purchasing new hair systems as the old ones wear out
- ✔ Changing your hair system to match your natural hair color as it changes due to aging (that is, as it turns gray)

In the end, there's no set cost for a hair system, and as long as you choose to wear one, you'll be paying something for it on a frequent or regular basis.

Assessing your psychological costs

You may wonder what psychological costs could possibly result from wearing a hair system. For some people, worrying constantly about their hair — Is it going to stay in place? Can other people tell they're wearing hair systems? Are people secretly laughing behind their backs? — may outweigh any benefit of having a full head of hair.

The only one who knows how you react to such things is you. If you know you're a worrier and are likely to spend much of your time reaching up to see if your hair's still there, or constantly trying to read strangers' expressions to catch their reactions to your system, you may be better off without a hair replacement system. Other options are available, after all; we cover them in Parts IV and V of this book.

Beware the wig salesman who wants to clip your hair!

Twenty-one-year-old Charlie was concerned about his frontal corner recession (the hair in the corners of his hairline meets the side hair of the temple), so he looked through the phone book and found a full page ad proclaiming a modern form of hair replacement and a medical breakthrough. Charlie got the courage to visit the company's office, where he met a likeable salesman who looked at Charlie's balding area and, with hardly a word, clipped the front of Charlie's frontal hairline back 2 inches from the front! "Don't worry about a thing," said the salesman. "If you don't like what I've got, there's no charge and you can just walk away."

Needless to say Charlie was freaked out with the frontal 2 inches of hair clipped close to the skin; his 3-inch-long hair behind it made for an embarrassing contrast. The salesman took out a small hair system with tape on the back and stuck it to the newly clipped area on Charlie's scalp. Immediately, Charlie had a full head of hair, but he was left with no choice but to buy the hair system. When he walked out of the office, although he felt okay about his new 'do, he was uncomfortable at having been taken in by the sales process.

This was the beginning of Charlie's 20-year relationship with hair systems. His hair system changed as his hair style changed, and as his hair grayed so did his hair system. As his balding progressed over time, his hair system became larger. The problem that Charlie didn't notice initially was that his hair systems were slowly pulling out the rest of his frontal hair. His hair system became an addiction, costing him thousands of dollars every year. Unfortunately, at no time was Charlie given the opportunity to explore other hair loss treatment options — he was hooked.

Considering the possibility of accelerated hair loss

Some hair systems accelerate hair loss. This is generally due to the attachment method causing traction on the existing hair. Glues and tapes are notorious for accelerating hair loss. Some doctors also theorize that the psychological stress of wearing the hair system (refer to the previous section) can contribute to hair loss. This theory has been observed in identical twins when one has a hairpiece and the other doesn't.

Dr. Rassman had a pair of identical twins in their late 20s. One had a hair system and the other did not. The one with the hair system used clips, but his hair loss had advanced far more than his identical twin brother who wore no hair system. Dr. Rassman has seen this in a number of identical twins.

Maintaining Your New Hair

Using a hair replacement system is much more complicated than simply buying something and sticking it on your head. (That only works if you're using your new hair to block the sun and not as a way to improve your appearance!) You've probably seen people with hair replacement systems that are so obvious — and so badly in need of TLC — that they turn you off the idea of a hair system. But you need to remember that a well-maintained and well-fitted system *isn't* noticeable. In order to help you achieve the best, unnoticeable results, this section covers some dos and don'ts for keeping your hair looking as good as the rest of you.

Staying active — and keeping your hair on!

If you're very active or participate in sports, one of your main concerns may be how difficult it will be to keep your hair in place while you're in the water or running down the soccer field, for example. Most people with hair systems try not to push them to the limits, at least not when other people are around!

Most wearers restrict many activities like water-skiing, yet many hair replacement advertisements show men wearing their products while water-skiing! We've heard reports from some people who have done just what the ads suggest and had their systems come off in the most embarrassing social situations. Our recommendation is that you use common sense, and if you think your hair system may not hold up to your activity, consider changing your plans.

Everyone is different, so what works for one person may not work for another. Generally, hair systems hold up to gentler sports (such as running, golf, tennis, most aerobic exercises and gym activities, and skiing the bunny slopes, for example), but if you're into more aggressive athletics, you may be better off taking off your hair system and wearing a hat instead. For example, direct contact sports are clearly risky for detachment.

Two other problems plague many hair system users:

- ✔ What to do when your system gets wet in the rain
- ✔ How to manage sweating underneath the hair system

Unfortunately, these problems aren't easily solved. Our best rec-ommendation is that you carry a spare hair system with you and make a switch when such problems occur.

Keeping up with regular care and maintenance

Many women — and men — have standing appointments at the hair or nail salon. Think of maintenance for your hair system in the same way — as just part of your normal routine. Following are some handy guidelines for the care of your hair system:

✔ **Set up a schedule for having your hair system washed — whether you do it yourself or take it to a professional.** Don't wait until it starts to smell.

- If you use a hair system that attaches with either clips or tapes, smell the system when you remove it at night. You should wash it frequently enough to keep any odor neu-tral and to avoid the "What's that smell?" look from your closest friends.

- If your hair system is attached with glue, and you're not an expert on the application of the glue, you may not be aware of a developing odor because you don't remove the hair system nightly. Therefore, your maintenance schedule should take into account the timing of develop-ing odors. Ask someone near and dear to you to give it a sniff and judge if your hair system needs to be washed. If you're too embarrassed to involve another person, just arrange a standing appointment with your system main-tenance service people.

✔ **If you have a weave, the weave will loosen as your hair grows, so you should have it professionally adjusted two or three times a month.** The longer you wait between adjusting the weave, the looser it will become. And the looser is becomes, the greater the risk of traction alopecia (refer to Chapter 5). A wig that moves around your head is not only uncomfortable, but you also have to worry that others may detect it because most people's hair doesn't shift around!

✔ **If your hair system involves wefts, you should have it serv-iced before the wefts come loose from the base of the hair that they're attached to.** It's relatively easy to feel the point of attachment, and when the wefts start to come off, you'll feel them peeling away. Servicing a weft requires expertise, and it's usually done by salons that specialize in this type of hair system. It's best to be proactive in servicing your weft and not wait for it to peel off; there's almost nothing more obvious than a weft that hangs apart from your hair and scalp.

✔ **Think of your hair system maintenance like you do car maintenance: Attend to it regularly, and have the whole system looked over for potential problems.** Your service experts will tell you when your hair system is wearing out, and if that's detected early, the repairs hopefully won't break the bank.

✔ **Don't forget to maintain your spare hair system(s).** It's always smart to be prepared for the unexpected, and you never know when you'll need your backup plan.

As you can see, the timing of your maintenance program depends largely on the type of hair system you have, but you'll always benefit from being proactive. For example, servicing your system before you take a vacation is a good move. With some experience under your belt, you'll figure out just how much preventive maintenance is required. Setting up a schedule is critical.

Recognizing when it's time to replace

Even the most expensive hair system won't last forever. On average, you can expect your system to last for a year or two with proper care. The more expensive hair systems made of human hair will last longer. As we mention earlier in this chapter, you'll need to replace your hair system as your natural hair color changes in order to keep the transition as seamless as possible. And if you work in sandy or dusty environments, it will become dirty, picking up dirt and grime between the hair filaments and in the foundation. The more dirt and grime on the hair system, the harder it is to clean (which may mean gentle washing isn't very effective) and the more frequently it requires washing.

Consider wearing a hat instead of your hair system when you're working in a dusty environment. It makes no difference if you're an executive who only occasionally visits construction sites — the hair system will pick up elements of the environments you visit, and that can either accelerate damage or be a tip-off to others that your hair's not really yours.

Chapter 7

Shopping for Hair Replacement Systems

*W*ith all the options today to seed, replant, or clone hair (just kidding about that last one — for now), you may wonder why you should consider a wig. Many people consider wigs, or the more modern term, hair replacement systems, because they're fearful of surgery or can't afford hair transplant surgery, or because they only need to cover temporary hair loss as with chemotherapy.

In this chapter, we talk about how wigs are made and measured, how to find the right wig for you, and how to care for it. We also explain how to tell a good wig from a bad one.

Getting Wiggy with It

When deciding to cover up your balding or thinning hair with a hair replacement system such as a wig, you may be leery because of the number of jokes made over the years about "bad rugs" and the cartoons illustrating wigs landing in someone's soup, or blowing across the parking lot.

Rest assured: Modern hair systems can be can be completely undetectable — and are well anchored, so that gaffes of the past can be completely avoided.

Don't be misled by the term "wig" into thinking that we're just discussing cover-ups for women; men's toupees and hairpieces are also considered wigs, or hair replacement systems.

Going Shopping: Where to Start?

For the most part, specialty shops such as wig makers aren't part of most people's daily shopping routine. So where do you start when you're looking for a hair replacement system — the yellow pages, the Internet, or by following someone with a good-looking wig and asking them where they bought it?

 The wig market has expanded greatly in the last few years, particularly in Asia, and is now a billion-dollar business. So lots of companies are competing for your business, and being a careful consumer can get you the best product at the best price. But before you start shopping, you've got to know how to do your research first.

Deciding which wig fits your needs and budget

Not surprisingly, your biggest consideration before shopping for a wig should be price for the initial purchase and in finding out the long-term cost to maintain it. A wig is expensive, and even good ones need replacing every year or two.

 You may also want a "hair and a spare" for times when you want a different hairstyle, or as a back up if something happens to the one you have.

The price of the wig depends on its quality and on what it's made of. The most common wigs are made of the following materials:

✔ **Human hair:** Wigs made of human hair are the highest quality and the most natural looking (and feeling). They usually start at around $1,200, and maintenance costs average a comparable amount per year.

✔ **Animal hair:** A wig made of goat or horsehair is a popular, cheaper alternative (in the low hundreds of dollars). Wigs are also made from other animals' hair, such as yak. These wigs also require maintenance similar to that of natural human hair.

✔ **Synthetic materials:** This is the cheapest option — such wigs are available for around $50. Wigs made of synthetic materials are the easiest to care for because the color and shape last longer. However, these wigs are also the least natural to the touch and eye.

✔ **Combination of human hair and synthetic materials:** Wigs often consist of both human hair and synthetic materials. The downside is that human hair needs to be maintained differently than the synthetic fibers.

The price of a wig also depends on whether it's been hand- or machine-made. For more on hand-made wigs, see the section "Understanding How a Custom-Fit Wig Is Made" later in this chapter.

✔ **Machine-made wigs:** This is the cheaper option. Strands of hair are sewn into a net base singularly or in groupings tied to a netting. They look very realistic when the hair falls in the style in which it was sewn, but if the wind blows or you pull the hair up, the netting below can be very visible and obvious. These wigs are normally used for costume parties rather than as hair replacement systems.

✔ **Hand-made wigs:** These wigs are more expensive and more realistic-looking. Each strand is sewn individually rather than in strips to make the hair fall and move more naturally — in fact, you can style hand-made wigs as you do your own hair.

Remember that the real cost of a wig made of human hair can add up to a few thousand dollars a year when you weigh in the purchase, replacement, and maintenance costs. You may also want to have your wig washed at the shop, because shop equipment probably can do a more thorough job of it than you can, and careful washing and drying can help extend the life of your hair system.

Finding a specialty shop

After you've determined how much you plan to spend, you have a better idea of where to shop. Some specialty shops may simply be out of your price range, but you never know until you ask. If you know someone who wears a hair replacement system, that person may be able to recommend a shop in your area. But if all your friends are skittish about discussing what's on top of their heads (a common problem for the new wig candidate), you may have to resort to opening the phone book and calling around. Look under both "Hair Replacement" and "Wigs" for shops near you.

Most specialty shops have full services, from sales to fitting and repairs all under one roof. Salespeople who are skilled and knowledgeable about the various products they sell generally work at the stores, but remember that they're still, first and foremost, salespeople who have a product to sell. Ask the following questions before you sign on the dotted line:

- How long has this shop been in business?

- Is the owner of the shop here? What's his background in replacement?

- How long have you (salesperson) worked here?

- Do you have any references I can talk to?

- What are the total costs, including fitting and adjustment costs?

- How often will I need maintenance on this product? (If the answer is "none," you're in the wrong shop! Every wig needs regular maintenance.)

- How long does a wig usually last? (If the answer is "forever," run! Most wigs last only a year or two.)

- What kind of materials do you use?

- What attachment systems do you use, and which ones do you recommend?

- Do you have a warranty? (In case hair starts falling off the minute you leave the shop)

- Are your wigs hand- or machine-made? Who makes them?

As with buying a car, you probably don't want to buy at the first shop you visit. Go to several specialty shops to get a better idea of the differences among shops and among their products. These are people you're going to be seeing often for styling and repairs, so if you don't feel comfortable in the shop, it's probably not a good choice for you.

Don't be talked into having any part of your head shaved in order to try a wig on, no matter what the salesperson tells you. Some sleazy facilities are very skilled in the art of the sale, and may try to get you to shave the front of your head so that you're stuck having to buy the wig just to keep from looking odd when you walk out the door.

Haircuts for wig wearers

One perk to wearing a wig is that getting a new style, even for an evening, is just a matter of getting a new wig. But most wig wearers still have some of their own hair underneath that still needs cutting and maintaining.

Do you take off your hair system for a hair cut or do you leave it in place? If your hair system is fixed on with clips, you can easily remove it to get your hair cut, but if you use glues to hold it in place, the hair cut can become a challenge. Often, the scalp is shaved under the hair system, but even hair buried under a wig continues to grow, and will eventually need a trim. If you want you hair cut around your wig, be sure the person cutting your hair knows how to manage your wig.

Fortunately, many wig shops offer haircuts as part of the services they supply their clients. Be sure and ask if your shop provides this service.

Choosing a style

Choosing a new hairstyle can be a bewildering task. Should you go radically different from your current color and style and buy something that looks like you magically woke up one morning with a new full head of hair? Or should you go for a gradual increase of hair and buy several wigs, each one a little fuller than the last, so no one will notice?

In general, you should choose a wig in the same way you choose a hairstyle: it should be a color that suits your skin tone and a style that suits your face shape. A stylist or wig salesperson can help you find the right style.

Buying online: Worth the risk?

Combine the popularity of hair replacement systems with the popularity of the Internet and what have you got? A lot of online options for ordering instant hair! But online sales don't give you that warm fuzzy feeling that any manufacturing or fitting problems will be taken care of. That's why most people seek a personalized service at a local wig salon when purchasing a hair system.

An Internet search for "hair replacement systems" returns hundreds of thousands of possibilities! The advantage to Internet shopping is mainly the cheaper cost and the extra privacy. You can choose a design, fill out and send the special forms for fitting requirements, and finalize the sale in a matter of minutes. Of course, experience taking measurements and buying off the

Internet may be difficult if you're a novice. And then when it comes in the mail, what do you do with it? How do you attach it? Does it feel custom made for your head? Very doubtful!

If you can't try a wig's fit before buying, try sizing your head by trying on a series of baseball caps and matching them up with wig sizes. Many of the wigs come in a series of standard sizes ranging from small to extra-large, so you may increase your chances of ordering a better fit if you have some idea of where you fall in that spectrum.

However, the old adage about getting what you pay for is definitely a factor in Internet shopping. Among the caveats of shopping online are the following:

- ✔ You don't know much about the people you're buying from. The Internet businesses come and go, and getting shafted is unfortunately not all that unusual when dealing with Internet companies that have to turn high volumes of sales.

- ✔ You can't see what you're buying in advance; materials used in wigs vary greatly, and cheap materials look just that: cheap.

- ✔ You may not measure your head correctly; an ill-fitting hair- piece is the biggest giveaway that your hair isn't your own.

- ✔ Corrections and adjustments are difficult; a local shop is much better at fixing problems as they occur. Internet trans- actions start to seem less convenient if you can't get anyone to answer your e-mails or calls.

- ✔ You still need to find someone locally to style, wash, or main- tain your hairpiece, unless you really want to send your hair back and forth through the mail.

Make sure you have a way to contact the Internet shop if you have problems. Do they have an 800 number? A hotline? E-mail that's answered frequently?

The dying art of wig making

Things have certainly changed in the wig making business over the past three cen- turies. The art of wig making, a growing and thriving trade in the 17th through 19th centuries, is being replaced by low-cost labor and mechanization. For years, wig making was a craft that took decades to learn and perfect. But like many trades- men skills of old, the economics of mass production are killing what's left of the old, personalized wig making business and the skills that went along with it.

Choosing a Human Hair Wig

If you decide on a human hair wig, be sure you know how to differentiate between the quality of the hair used and the way in which the wig was made. The variables that dictate the quality of the wig include the following:

- **Thickness of the hair:** Thick hairs are usually less expensive but cover better; finer hairs, which don't provide as much cover for each strand of hair used, are more natural in appearance and softer to the touch. Wigs made of finer human hair require more hair to provide adequate cover, which, of course, increases the cost, because the more hair used, the greater the labor and the time required to build the wig. The hair needs to be dense enough to prevent light from penetrating through it, into the netting, and down to the scalp.

  Using three or four fine hairs combined together may increase the thickness of the hair and reduce the cost of labor, but it doesn't feel as delicate as when single strands of hair are used and appropriately knotted in position. Animal hair (such as horse or goat hair) is popular among some wig makers to keep costs down because these hairs are thicker and less hair is needed to fill out the wig.

- **Method of hair attachment:** Each hair is either glued to the foundation (a process more common in cheaper wigs) or sewn into the mesh one hair at a time (a technique more common in quality wigs).

- **Type of knotting:** The number and style of knots used to attach the hair contribute to the security of the hair fixation to the mesh. Single strands of hair with single knots tend to loosen and come apart; these wigs don't hold up well over time. Single strands of fine human hair with multiple knots are more secure. The type of knots and the stitch techniques that are used are critically important.

  Sometimes, three or four hairs are tied together at the base, which reduces the labor cost. More hair tied at the base may be visible on close inspection.

If each individual hair is fine human hair placed one by one in high density and knotted with at least two knots to secure it to the mesh, the wig becomes a quality product that looks and feels more natural.

It may sound odd, but to get some insight into wig making, go to a carpet store and ask to see the rugs that they sell. Ask the salesperson to tell you the difference between a fine expensive carpet and a cheap one. He or she will almost certainly tell you about the number of stitches per inch, the quality of the fibers he is using (wool or silk quality), the type of wool or synthetics used, the number of knots per strand, and so on.

Choosing a Synthetic Wig

A handmade human hair wig may not be in your budget at the moment, but if the thought of a synthetic wig makes you cringe, you may be surprised when you do a little shopping around! Synthetic wigs are more natural-looking than ever before. The synthetics are most frequently made of a monofilament, somewhat like a piece of fishing line. These come in many sizes and colors and can be sewn into the foundation mesh. They don't hold the knots well, so more knots must be used. Popular monofilaments include Kanekalon and Toyokalon.

The advantages of going synthetic include the following:

- ✔ It's yours the day you buy it; you don't have to wait for your new hair to be custom made.
- ✔ You can see exactly what you're getting.
- ✔ It's relatively inexpensive.
- ✔ You can change your look by buying several different wigs without breaking the bank.

The disadvantages of a synthetic wig include some of the following considerations:

- ✔ It doesn't look as natural as human hair.
- ✔ You can't style it.
- ✔ You can't get it fitted specifically to your head.
- ✔ It may feel plastic to the touch.
- ✔ Depending upon the foundation and any stitching, close inspection may reveal your secret.

Synthetics don't accept a perm, and the color can't be changed to any significant degree. Synthetic wigs are designed to stay looking the way they did when you originally bought them; trying to change or restyle them can cause significant damage to the wig. The life of a good synthetic wig can be one or two years or more, depending on their quality, how well you take care of them, and how often you wash them. Synthetic materials are fairly sturdy and are likely to last longer than human hair wigs.

Understanding How a Custom-Fit Wig Is Made

The foundation of a custom-made wig starts with a fabric mesh cut to the head size of the wearer. The foundation is usually a large size polyester-cotton-type lace fitted over a wig-block and cut according to, the penciled outline. The master wig maker then pins a finer lace to the front and to the back of the foundation while holding the leading edges with pins (see Figure 7-1). The mesh foundation is pinned to a block, and the wig maker places individual hairs into the mesh one at a time. Each hair is knotted so that the direction of the hair is controlled.

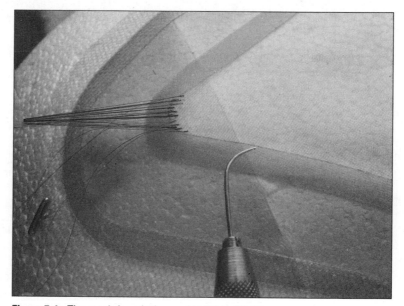

Figure 7-1: The mesh foundation and individual hairs.

Measuring for a wig

The fit of a wig does a lot to enhance its overall appearance and realistic look. Think of a customized suit of clothes that accounts for your uniquely sized shoulders and waist. Humans just don't come in standardized sizes. When you measure for a wig, the measurer holds a cloth measuring tape snug to the scalp, keeping the tape flat to avoid twists and kinks in the tape. Expect the following areas of measurement:

✔ The circumference from your proposed hairline to the back most prominent part of the skull, keeping it about ½ inch above the ears.

✔ The lowest rear point of the skull in the middle (just before the place where the bend in the neck can be felt when you tilt your head back) to the top of your forehead.

✔ From ear to ear with the tape going over the top of the head.

✔ From ear to ear with the tape going across the forehead.

✔ From the temple prominence to the very back of the head. The *temple prominence* should be at a line equal to the upper arch of your eyebrows and is generally located approximately 1½ inches from the side border of the eyebrow.

The wig maker then cuts the mesh foundations to these measurements.

Remember that the head is oval or round, and the mesh foundation is flat. Like a map of the world, the curves must be created from the flat mesh.

Less expensive wigs have a stretchable foundation, with the size chosen so that one wig size may fit many head sizes. More expensive wigs are customized, so you can choose the color, hair length, hair texture and style. Some wigs have Velcro strips inside them that the wearer can tighten for a better fit, much like the belt on your pants.

Most wig sales facilities have a variety of stock sizes (small, medium small, medium, medium large, and large), from which your wig can be fit to your head (like fitting a suit from a fine haberdasher). This fitting process is a clear advantage over an Internet purchase, where you can't feel and see the product as it may appear on your head.

Sound complicated? At least it helps explain why custom wigs are better, yet so much more expensive, than wigs off the rack.

Tools of the trade

As with every trade, wig making requires a particular set of tools. The basic tools are as follows:

✔ **A punch needle:** This is the needle used to attach the hair to the wig's base. The traditional punch was just a sawed off sewing needle, but it was hard to push through a latex or silicone pad. A properly designed punch needle has a hook near the tip of the needle, making it possible to just push the needle through a latex edge, grab a hair or a group of hairs and pull it back through the mask.

✔ **Nylon or polyester lace:** A very fine, skin-colored lace made of nylon or polyester is used at the periphery of a quality wig that is attached to the central foundation. Figure 7-2 shows a very expensive wig with a lace front.

A full range of colors for the mesh is necessary because of the wide variety of skin colors found in the population. The mesh takes on the person's regular skin color so that the hair looks natural when parted, as in Figure 7-3.

✔ **Make-up brushes of varying sizes and textures:** Make-up brushes are used to refine the leading edge to match the skin tone in the final steps of the construction process. These brushes refine the final product stroke by stroke.

✔ **Styling tongs in various shapes and sizes:** Tongs help shape the hair to produce the desired hairstyle. The process of shaping and styling the human hair wigs is the same process used in salons for creating the style, shown in Figure 7-4.

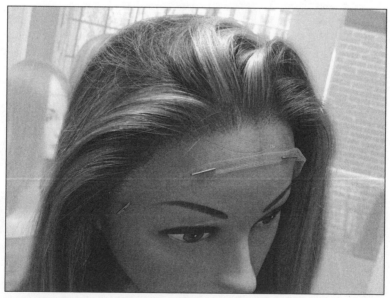

Figure 7-2: The leading edge of a very expensive wig.

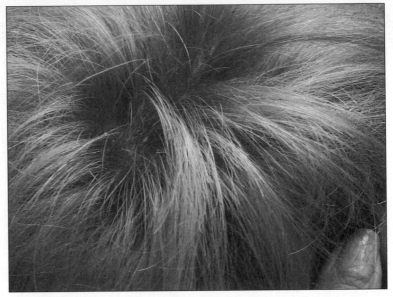

Figure 7-3: The scalp of an expensive wig looks very natural.

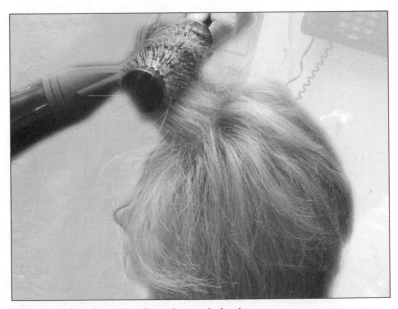

Figure 7-4: Shaping and styling a human hair wig.

Styles range widely from gentle wavy to more radical, ornamental hair styles. With the many options available, styling the wig is only limited by the imagination of the buyer and the creative skills of the wig maker, and the owner's input is critical in this part of the process.

Cosmetics help touch up the leading edge of the wig and blend the hair with the person's natural hair. Streaking a blonde or platinum color to individual hairs can add that touch of luxury to the styling.

Picking Up Your New Hair

You just got the call — your new hair has arrived! Nervous? Excited? Scared about being seen in public for the first time? These are all normal reactions as you open the package or head to the shop to pick up your new hair replacement system.

Trying it on for size

If you had your head measured at a specialty shop, your new hair probably fits like a glove after a few minor adjustments. If you bought online, the measurements you provided determine the final product's fit, and having adjustments done isn't going to be as easy.

Attaching your hair easily

You can attach your wig to your head in a number of ways; you can even have it grafted into your scalp! (We discuss specific ways to attach hair replacement systems in Chapter 6.) Practice makes perfect; be involved in attaching your wig even in the store so that you begin to get a feel for the process. Eventually, you'll be able to streamline your attaching routine.

Adjusting to wig wearing

Not everyone adjusts easily to wearing a hair replacement system. If your first day with your new hair leaves you feeling self-conscious and uncomfortable, you're not alone. You may hold your head funny because it feels unfamiliar on your head or walk more carefully because you're worried about disturbing your 'do'. You may even feel like people can sense your discomfort. Give yourself time to adjust; most new habits take time to adjust to, so be patient when it comes to getting comfortable with your new look.

If you aren't happy with your wig

If you're not comfortable with your new hair after a few days or weeks, try to figure out why. Consider the following questions:

✔ Is your hair system uncomfortable? Is it too hot, heavy, or itchy?

✔ Are you sweating too much?

✔ Is the adhesive or attachment that you're using uncomfortable?

✔ Are you self-conscious or worried about your wig falling off?

After you figure out exactly what's bothering you, go back to the specialty shop where you purchased it, or contact the shop if you bought it online. If it's a problem with comfort or the adhesive, you may be able to have the wig altered to correct the problem.

In a short time, the nerve endings on your scalp will get used to the feel of the wig on your head, and you won't even know you have it on. If you wear glasses, you may remember how difficult it was to adjust to them in the beginning; something on your head is just as hard to get used to at first.

As for self-consciousness, just give yourself time. Wearing a wig takes getting used to, like everything else.

Going Public with Your Hair

Walking out in public the first time with a new wig is a strange feeling. You may feel self-conscious, but don't fret — you and everyone else will be used to your new hair in no time, and in the end it will make you more confident rather than less.

✔ **Have an answer ready.** You're going to get questions if you've suddenly grown a new head of hair overnight! If you're the boss at your workplace, you may not get direct questions, but you can be sure you'll be the object of conversation! Consider beating everyone to the punch by bringing the topic up first.

✔ **Consider a holiday.** It may be easier to get away for a while and get used to wearing the wig around people who didn't know you before you wore it. This tactic can give you time to feel more comfortable and hence more confident about your new look. Confidence is ever-critical in whatever you decide.

Caring For Your Wig

A hair replacement system is no different than your own hair; it requires washing, styling, and sometimes even trimming. Your wig will stay natural looking if you care for it properly, and in the next sections, we tell you how.

Maintaining human hair wigs

You can style human hair wigs much like your natural hair, but they do require care. We recommend using only styling tools such as curling irons and rollers that are made specifically for wigs to avoid causing unnecessary damage to the wig.

When cleaning your wig, start by removing the wig (very carefully!) and any tangles with your fingers or a fine comb. Never apply force. You can gently remove any stains with a toothbrush and warm water. Wash the wig with shampoo, and always use conditioner afterward. Human hair wigs can be washed more often than synthetics, since their attachment to the mesh is more secure.

Never use a blow dryer or wring your wig dry. Always blot it with a towel and then place it on its stand to dry.

Maintaining synthetic wigs

As we mention earlier in the chapter, you really can't style or alter the color of a synthetic wig, so your main maintenance task is washing. How long you go between cleanings of your wig depends largely on your lifestyle and environment. For normal wear, a good rule of thumb to use is to wash and condition your wig every 15 to 20 uses or so.

If you work in an environment with more pollution, such as in a restaurant where you're exposed to kitchen grease or a place with a lot of cigarette smoke, you may want to wash your wig more often. You can also opt to have separate wigs for work and home. In any case, if you wash your wig more than once a week, it won't last long.

Remember, the nose knows, and if your wig doesn't smell fresh to you, it doesn't smell good to others around you either.

Washing and cleaning is an art form for all wigs, particularly the synthetic wig. Never use hot water — it can damage the synthetic fibers. Lukewarm water is okay. Soaking the wig for a short period of time and even using gentle steam may work, but don't let too much heat get to the wig.

Dry the wig with a towel. After it's somewhat dry, you can use a blow dryer, but very high heat settings can singe the edges, melt the synthetic fiber or the foundation, and crack the filaments. Hot rollers may also damage or melt the synthetic hair.

Wearing a Wig for Temporary Hair Loss

Wigs aren't just used by balding men and women with thinning hair. They can also be a valuable solution for people who have temporary hair loss as a result of some medical conditions (such as alopecia areata or cancer chemotherapy).

Dealing with a life-threatening illness is hard enough without having to worry about losing your hair too. Some people who know they're going to be taking drugs that cause hair loss find it less stressful to buy a wig before they start treatment. As soon as you start to feel uncomfortable about you hair falling out, you've got the wig handy.

Because hair loss caused by chemotherapy and other disease is often temporary, you may feel that a less expensive synthetic wig is adequate for your needs. Consider buying several to give yourself a lift when you're feeling down about your appearance.

Many insurance companies cover the cost of a wig used when hair loss is the result of chemotherapy. Your doctor will probably need to write a (carefully worded) letter to the insurance company requesting the benefit; most insurance companies don't cover the cost of a "wig" but do cover a "hair prosthesis" or "cranial hair prosthesis."

Some organizations recycle wigs for cancer patients at low or no cost. The American Cancer Society (www.cancer.org) may be able to provide you with the name of an organization near you.

Chapter 8

Concealing Hair Loss with Fibers, Sprays, and More

. . . .

. . . .

*W*ouldn't it be nice if you could thicken your hair with just the wave of a magic wand? Although we can't tell you how to pull a new head of hair out of a magician's hat, in this chapter we show you a few ways to pull some sleight of hand — or in this case, head — by applying products such as spray-on fibers and spray-on concealers and paint on masking products that give the illusion of more hair without resorting to the expense of hairpieces or hair transplants.

You do, however, need to have some existing hair for these concealers to work.

Styling Some Basic Hair "Thickening" Tricks

Before you start spraying your hair or painting your scalp, try some simple styling techniques to help conceal hair loss or thinning. For example, get rid of the old comb-over that only emphasizes your hair loss and try a shorter cut to give the illusion of more hair. Or just shave it all off so that it looks like bald is your choice and not the result of failing hair follicles.

Hair and skin color can also play a subtle role in achieving the appearance of fuller hair. A sharp contrast between the color of your hair and the color of your skin will accentuate a thinning hair line. You may not be thrilled with your graying hair, but gray hair actually blends your hair and skin tones well, which results in your hair appearing fuller.

The combination of blond hair and fair skin makes your hair look fuller than black hair and light skin. Many men and women choose to color their hair to a lighter or darker color to bring down the contrast between the hair and scalp color. Going blond is good, or consider a slow transition to a sandy hair color if you have a light skin tone. Platinum blond and glistening white hair reflect light, making it more difficult to see through the hair to the scalp. Proper use of hair dyes can produce such changes.

Keeping your hair shiny can help it appear fuller as well. The shine allows the hair to reflect light better, whereas dull hair allows you to see through to the scalp easier.

The added body of curls or waves in the hair can also help it appear fuller. Some men and women who have naturally straight hair perm it to achieve the appearance of more volume and fullness. Many women whose hair has begun thinning with age make their hair appear fuller by perming, teasing, and lightening it (all of which can cause damage; see Chapter 3 for more). Men are starting to go this route as well.

Hair shaft thickness also plays an important role in styling and imparting a fuller hair appearance. A coarse hair shaft provides more coverage than finer hair. There are many hair thickeners available and some shampoos and conditioners will also promote thickening. Other products such as hair wax, pomades, horse tail grooming products, and gels that can help your hair appear fuller (see Chapter 3 for more on products).

Fooling Around with Fibers

Feel like shaking some new hair onto your head? It may not be as good as the real thing, but topical products made of colored protein fibers can conceal hair thinning. These fibers, which come in pepper shaker-type bottles, adhere to bases of the hair follicles and the scalp, adding bulk to the hair shaft. See Figure 8-1.

These mostly stay in place by static electricity but fixing sprays are available that add more holding power. The results can be dramatic, and the process is quick and easy.

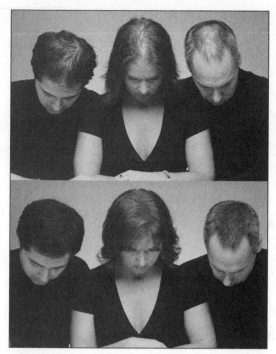

Figure 8-1: Fiber products cling to the scalp and existing hair to conceal balding areas.

Watching hair grow before your very eyes

There are many types of fiber products that can make hair shafts thicker; two of the more well-known products are Toppik and XFusion. These products are comprised of organic keratin fibers with a similar chemical makeup to human hair. You apply the product by spraying, painting, or sprinkling it on your scalp, where the fibers cling to your existing hair and create an illusion of a thicker and fuller hairline. The fibers stick to your existing hairs by static electricity, so you don't have to worry about it coming off.

After the product is on your hair and scalp, it's very difficult to take off completely — except with a thorough hair wash. See Figure 8-2 for an example of a fiber product at work.

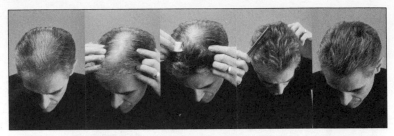

Figure 8-2: Before and after pictures with Toppik fibers.

Toppik and other hair fiber products should blend in with your own the hair color, so choose the right color for the best results. The subtle addition of the extra fibers will diminish any contrast between your hair and scalp color. The drastic improvement also comes from the fibers adhering to the fine vellus hairs — shorter hairs which have little or no pigment — which can make your hair look thicker. In all, it's a great illusion.

Apply the product before you put on a white shirt. And remember to comb through your hair to ensure the fibers are fixed firmly.

 How well these products work depends on how much natural hair you have to work with. They obviously won't work very well if you're bald or nearly bald with only a few hairs. In that case, a limited hair transplant can give you enough hair to use this product successfully. These products are excellent for making a hair transplant look fuller and may forestall more surgeries.

 The problem with most fiber concealers is that they may not work at the hairline, but with a template placed slightly behind where the thin hair starts, you can create a reasonable illusion of a frontal hairline. Both Toppik and Xfusion offer spray applicators which can be used with their hairline templates.

Facing the elements

Any time you apply something to your head, it's normal to worry about it coming off at an inopportune moment, which can lead to embarrassing situations.

Fiber products are pretty difficult to disengage (depending upon the manufacturer), with the following caveats:

> ✔ **A light rain won't affect fiber products because the fibers don't dissolve in water.** But getting caught in a monsoon and being literally drenched in water may be a different story.

> ✔ **Wind shouldn't affect the fiber concealer because static electricity keeps the fibers clinging to your existing hair.** However, we wouldn't stick our heads out of the car going 60 mph to test this theory, and you probably shouldn't either.

> ✔ **If you sweat heavily, some products will not run, while others may.** Try not to run your fingers through your hair in public (or let someone else do it!) if you're not confident in the product you are using; test your fiber concealer at home (rather than in public) to see just how far you can push it with a sweaty head or with your fingers running through your hair.

If you still worry that the fibers may shed or loosen and cause an embarrassing fallout, you can always use hair spray for that additional safety cushion.

Some 'fiberhold' products are made by the companies that make these concealer products just for that purpose. Practice with the product you choose so there'll be no surprises.

Making fiber cover ups part of your routine

The obvious point of using any form of applied concealer to mask baldness is that it's temporary. It may be a quick fix to your problem, but it's only a short-term solution to a long-term problem.

However, the sad reality about balding is that once it starts, the chances of returning to a full head of hair are almost nil. So when you start concealing your vanishing hair line, it's likely to be a part of your daily grooming routine for the rest of your life.

You may get to a point where you become addicted to the product because it can make such a dramatic difference in your appearance. Unlike other addictions, this one isn't a bad thing, really. The product can be miraculously undetectable as long as you have enough hair for the fibers to cling to.

However, as you go through the balding process and lose more hair, you may come to a point when the fibers may be visible to the discriminating eye. At that point, you may have to give up the fibers and deal with thin hair that looks even thinner because you no longer can use the fibers to conceal the thinning effectively. This is when it's a particularly good idea to look at alternatives.

As we mention earlier in this chapter, even a limited hair transplant can give you enough fibers to continue to use the product.

Taking the time to apply the product

One of the problems with fiber concealers is that they can be time consuming to use. Toppik, for example, boasts of a 30-second application time and when you become experienced with it, you may find that estimate to be accurate. But it doesn't include the time it takes to style your hair and wash out the fibers at the end of the day.

Whether you can apply Toppik in only 30 seconds is debatable because different people have different needs based on how much hair they currently have. Obviously, the less hair you have, the longer it will take to apply and the more important your skill in applying the product will be.

Spray-on Hair

Who doesn't remember those hair-in-a-can ads on TV in years past? Although those made-for-TV products were the butt of many jokes, the concept made sense.

The goal of many of these spray on solutions is to darken your scalp to the color of your hair and fill out your thinning hair to make your scalp disappear. The original products may have been laughable, but now there's a new generation of colored sprays. The best known is Fullmore. It uses aerosol propellant to spray tiny color-matched fibers that cling to your existing hair and darken your scalp.

Sprays are quick to use and offer probably the fastest way to camouflage large areas, but you need some hair to have them work well. On the downside, they're not as precise as dab-on concealers, and not quite as natural in appearance with keratin fibers like Toppik in an area with more natural hair still left.

You apply products like Fullmore by holding the spray can around eight inches from your head and spraying while moving the can around for an even result. Put a towel on your shoulders to avoid any overspray. The results are quick, if not quite as convincing as fibers.

Be careful when going out in the rain, as there is some run-off potential in downpours.

After application, you should apply a FiberHold Spray (designed to bond fibers to hair) or a good hair spray. Once sealed, the product won't flake or come off, and you can brush through it without worry. It will not blow out in the wind or run from perspiration. Like all other concealers, it washes out with vigorous shampooing.

Feeling like the real thing

Face it: As much as the chemical makeup of fiber concealers is similar to human hair, the actual feel and texture of fibers on your hair may not be the same as a real, thick, full head of hair. Fibers tend to be finer than human hair, which can lead to flyaway hairs under certain conditions (which you should test in private; see the earlier section, "Facing the elements").

You may be self-conscious about how the fibers look and feel on your head and therefore constantly worry about your hair. And heaven forbid if someone you're dating wants to run their fingers through your fibrous hairs — be very careful about that no touch zone!

Applying Foundation

Using a fiber concealer to add fullness to your remaining hair still leaves you with another problem: covering your hairless scalp. If you're an artist, you may have contemplated painting a hair scene on your balding head. Fortunately, you don't have to be artistic to apply foundation makeup made specifically to cover shiny bald skin and blend the scalp color with the hair color.

Coloring your head

Foundations that conceal hair loss are best compared to women's cosmetic foundation or pressed powder. Essentially, foundation for your scalp is created from coloring and emollients (moisturizers) and is applied in much the same way that foundation is applied to the face.

What foundation does is conceal the whiter or lighter parts of your scalp. This masks your hairline, making it look as though your hair isn't thinning because the scalp coloring is brought closer to your hair color.

Like fiber concealers, scalp foundation will only work to conceal thinning hair if you have hair in the area to begin with. This material can't be used on the hairline to address your hairline problems; the hairline is a separate beast you have to deal with.

Using a sponge applicator, you simply shade in parts of your scalp where your hairline is thinning.

Accepting the limitations

One of the problems with foundation products is that they don't add fullness to your actual hair like fiber products do. However, foundations do reduce the visibility of the scalp through what hair you have, and this effect may work well if you just have minor thinning. But if you have a relatively large area that needs covering, a foundation may leave you with an imbalance of hair to scalp ratio. Hair systems (see Chapter 7) or hair transplants may be the only option for those without enough hair.

Using a foundation can actually expose your thinning hair (at least to yourself) because a close look in a good light, like the bathroom, may reveal the painted-on look between the hairs.

You can combine foundation products with fiber concealers, thereby tackling both the hair and the scalp imbalance. This works when the amount of hair that you have isn't quite enough for the fiber sprays. The foundation darkens the scalp enough so that it doesn't show through after you use the fiber sprays like Toppik to thicken the hair that you still have.

Taking the time to paint

As with fiber concealers, foundations can take some time to apply. You may find it easier to apply over a wider area, painting with broad strokes, but precision control of specific spots may be more difficult. If you use a fiber in combination with the foundation, then the foundation should be laid down first.

The hair you have is always styled after you apply the foundation and before the fibers are used. Many foundation users find that they don't have to put it on every day. Some of the products may even last through a shampoo.

Scalp foundations are a temporary fix to a long-term problem. Certainly, masking and concealing something that may be a source of insecurity is one way of coping with the problem at hand. However, you should keep in mind that there's no longevity to this solution; you have to do it again every day or every other day, depending upon your own situation.

Comparing Cover-ups

Many hair loss concealing products, whether they're powder-based or fiber-based, perform similar functions, so how do you choose the right solution for you? Table 8-1 lays it all out for you, comparing features of three products on the market.

Many people use combinations of the various products, either in different areas or together in the same area. We recommend that you try all the products to find the right product.

Table 8-1   Comparison of Popular Concealing Products

Features	COUVRé	Toppik	DermMatch	FULLMORE
Type and application	Foundation; dab on	Fiber; shake or spray on	Foundation; dab on	Fiber; spray on
Masks the scalp	Yes	Yes	Yes	Yes
Neutralizes scalp shine	Yes	Yes	Yes	Yes
Builds the hair	Base only	Throughout the hair	Base only	Base Only
Undetectable	Yes somewhat	Yes very	Yes somewhat	Somewhat
Number of colors available	8	8	8	8
Covers gray	Yes	Yes	Yes	Yes
Lasts through sweat, rain, and wind	Yes	Yes	Yes	Yes
Lasts through swimming	Yes	No	Somewhat	Yes
Easy to shampoo out	Yes	Yes	Yes	Yes
Lasts until shampooed out	Yes	Yes	Yes	Yes
Apply to damp or dry hair and Scalp	Either	Dry hair and Scalp Only	Damp hair is better	Dry Hair and Scalp Only

(continued)

Table 8-1 *(continued)*

Can be applied precisely to scalp	Yes	Yes Covers Broader area	Yes Covers Broader area	Covers Area
Time needed for typical application	2 minutes	30 seconds	2 minutes	30 seconds
Effective for very front of hairline	No Yes	Yes	Yes	No
Finishing spray recommended	No	Yes	No	Yes
Safe to use after a hair transplant	Yes	Yes	Yes	Wait 2 weeks
FDA-approved ingredients	Yes	Yes	Yes	Yes

Trying Thickeners

Do hair thickeners work? Yes, they do! But their effects are only temporary, and they have some limitations. Some men who are thinning use wax and pomade to make their hair look fuller. These products are the same as those that were so popular in the 1950s when the popular style for young men was slicked back hair.

In addition to achieving the slick look, these products also add extra thickness to your hair and provide the feeling and appearance of fullness.

A thicker hair shaft increases the fullness of one's hair exponentially. Even small increments of added thickness can have a major impact on the fullness of the hair (refer to the section, "Fooling Around with Fibers," earlier in this chapter for products that increase hair shaft fullness). Doubling the thickness of a single hair will increase the overall bulk fourfold. So, thickening each and every hair shaft may produce four times more bulk than having more hair!

Medications such as Propecia works so well for much the same reason. Propecia not only has the potential to grow new hair, but it also thickens tiny miniaturized hair to provide more coverage. You can read more about drugs such as Propecia in Chapter 9.

Some shampoos and conditioners can also make your hair look thicker by leaving a thin film of nutrients and oils on each hair strand. The film makes each hair fiber look shiny and healthy, which certainly can give your hair bounce and a feeling of fullness.

Some products also hydrate the hair shafts, adding increments of volume to them as they swell from absorbing water. But these products have limitations when your hair is thinning and you don't have enough to build upon as a foundation.

In short, the hair thickeners don't provide the dramatic results of fiber and powder concealers. Hair thickeners work best if you have very early thinning and lots of thinner hairs.

Using Concealers after a Hair Transplant

The impact of concealing agents can be remarkable, but they don't work in a bald frontal area or places where there's just not enough hair to work with. If you decide on a hair transplant to supply some needed hair, the concealing agents can work for a lifetime because the hair from a hair transplant lasts a lifetime.

Concealers that darken the scalp work well with transplants even if there's either not enough hair or enough money to cover the whole head with transplanted hair. Figure 8-3 shows a man who would have been completely bald had he not had hair transplants. Unfortunately, he didn't have enough donor hair to get the fullness he wanted, so he applied a concealing foundation to his scalp.

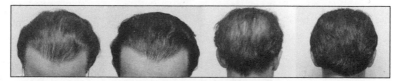

Figure 8-3: Top view of a post-transplant patient without (a) and with concealer (b); back view without (c) and with concealer (d).

Note that the see-through appearance in the first and third pictures in Figure 8-3 show the thinning that the concealer masks in the second and fourth pictures. The hair transplant gave this patient his frontal hairline back, and with concealers and a combed back hairstyle that gives the illusion of more hair he has achieved his hair restoration goal and is a happy camper with minimal inconvenience.

Combinations of hair thickeners, hair fibers, scalp coloring, and hair transplants can contribute greatly to achieving the goals of an illusion of hair when, in fact, the hair isn't all there.

Part IV
Pharmaceutical, Laser, and Topical Therapies

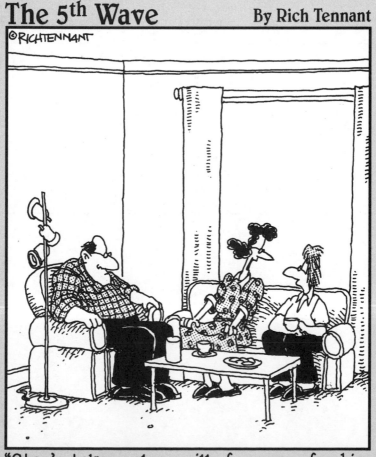

"Stan's taken salmon pills for years for his hair loss. Other than an urge to swim upstream each Fall, he hasn't experienced any side effects."

In this part . . .

*H*air loss therapy is a booming business, and there's no shortage of pills and topical potions, not to mention laser treatments, to help your hair grow. In this section, we look at what's on the market, both the good and the bad; we also consider more natural options, including eating your way to healthy hair.

Chapter 9

Turning to Prescription Medications for Hair Loss

. . . .

In This Chapter

▶ Being realistic about what drugs can do

▶ Keeping DHT in check with finasteride and dutasteride

▶ Targeting hair follicles with minoxidil

▶ Checking out some additional medications for women

. . . .

*T*ake a pill, grow your hair back. Sounds like a winning arrangement, doesn't it? Unfortunately, although a few prescription medications can help with specific types of hair loss, the magic hair pill has yet to be invented.

In this chapter, we look at prescription drugs that help with hair loss, drugs that may help some people some of the time (and that may include you), and drugs that are of no help whatsoever.

Managing Expectations

People generally expect miracles from prescription medications, and medications touted for hair loss are no exception. It's important to recognize the capabilities and limitations of medical treatments for hair loss therapies before you start using one. What topical (the ones you pour on your head) and oral drugs can do is stop hair loss in some people and sometimes regrow hair in areas that aren't yet totally bald. What they can't do is regrow all the hair you've lost.

Hair that you lost many years ago isn't likely to start growing. If you're satisfied with the idea of stopping hair loss and perhaps experiencing some mild regrowth, then you may be very happy with the results of taking some medications. But if you expect to regain the flowing locks you had in your teens, then you're sure to be disappointed.

Be patient when starting pharmaceutical hair loss treatment. Results take many months, not days or weeks. You must commit to treatment for at least one year to know if you're truly going to see any real benefit for pharmaceutical treatment. Remember, hair grows slowly, and it will take a considerable amount of time before you notice a difference.

Always use the medication as prescribed — whether that's once daily, twice a day, or what ever regime your doctor prescribes for the best possible chance of results. If you stop using the medicine, you can expect to lose all the hair that you may have gained from this therapy as well as any hair you would have lost while you were on the therapy, but luckily not more. After about six months your hair will look as if you'd never used the medication, and you'll resume losing hair at your natural rate.

The thought of taking a pill or using a solution on your scalp daily forever may seem discouraging. However, we encourage patients not to think of it that way. You can always decide at some point in the future that hair isn't as important to you as it once was and stop using the medicine.

In addition, it's possible that the future will bring better treatments for hair loss and perhaps a permanent cure. People use medication regularly for all kinds of conditions, such as high blood pressure or cholesterol, and it just becomes part of the daily routine. In time, the same is true with hair loss prescription medication.

Inhibiting DHT with Finasteride (Propecia)

One of the few prescription medications that really works to replace hair lost from male pattern baldness is finasteride, more commonly known as Propecia. Here we describe why it works and for whom; we also get into some of the side effects and the pros and cons of taking the drug so that you can make an informed decision with your doctor.

The discovery of finasteride

There's a common misconception that finasteride was first conceived as a prostate medication and was coincidentally found to prevent hair loss. The reality is that in 1974, researchers described a group of male children from the Dominican Republic who were deficient in the enzyme 5-alpha reductase (5AR). These male children had very low levels of DHT, and throughout their lives, their prostates remained small and they didn't develop male pattern hair loss or acne.

The scientists' goal was to find a drug that could block the 5AR enzyme and mimic the abnormality found in these boys. The scientists then could use this drug to prevent both prostate enlargement and hair loss. A deliberate (business) decision was made to seek Food and Drug Administration (FDA) approval for its use in treating prostate enlargement (a medical condition) rather than hair loss (a cosmetic problem).

In 1992, 5 mg finasteride was released under the brand name Proscar for use in men over 50 with prostate enlargement. Some men taking Proscar noted hair growth in balding or bald areas of their scalps. Scientific studies were done to determine if this drug would reduce the balding process and possibly grow hair. Varying doses of finasteride were tested to determine the safest and most effective dose for the treatment of hair loss, and in 1997, the FDA approved finasteride 1 mg per day (Propecia) for the treatment of male pattern baldness.

How finasteride works

As we explain in Chapter 4, male pattern baldness (androgenetic alopecia in medical lingo) is caused by the effects of the male hormone dihydrotestosterone (DHT) on genetically susceptible hair follicles predominantly in the front, top, and crown of the scalp (not the back and sides).

DHT causes hair loss by shortening the growth phase of the hair cycle, which leads to a decreased size (thickness) or miniaturization of the follicles. The affected hair grows more slowly or stops growing completely and progressively evolves into a shorter and finer hair until it eventually disappears.

Two of the male sex hormones are testosterone and dihydrotestosterone (DHT). Cells in the body metabolize testosterone and turn it into DHT. The traffic cop that supervises this process is an enzyme called 5-alpha reductase (5AR). The two types of 5AR are

✔ **Type I** is located mainly in sebaceous (sweat) glands, keratinocytes, and fibroblasts. Its exact role in hair growth has not been determined. This enzyme catalyzes the conversion of testosterone into androstenedione (another hormone) which seems to be related to the production of sebum. The role of Type II 5AR in hair loss is not well defined.

✔ **Type II** is found in the skin and the sheath of hair follicles on the scalp. This form of the enzyme seems to cause hair loss in those with the gene for hair loss, and can be blocked by the actions of drugs like finasteride.

The drug finasteride makes 5AR work less effectively, reducing the body's ability to produce DHT. When you take the drug orally, it reaches the bloodstream and the scalp hair follicles, where it decreases the amount of DHT made in the hair follicles.

Finasteride at the 1 milligram per day dose has been clinically shown to decrease serum DHT levels by almost 70 percent. Although many professionals falsely think that finasteride lowers a man's testosterone level, in fact, on average finasteride causes a rise in serum testosterone levels by 9 percent, although this is still within the normal range.

Testing the efficacy of finasteride

Propecia is the brand name for finasteride at the 1 mg dose, and it's proven to be very effective in the treatment of common pattern hair loss. Studies have shown that after five years of treatment, almost half of men treated with Propecia demonstrated an increase in hair growth, and 90 percent of men maintained most of their hair in previous thinning areas over this time period. Only 10 percent were rated as having lost hair when compared to their baseline hair measurements. In those not taking the drug, 75 percent were rated as having lost hair during the course of the study.

One mg finasteride can help you to preserve the hair you've got at any age, but it works best for hair regrowth in younger patients or those who have had recent hair loss in the past two to three years. Occasionally, people over age 50 see regrowth of some hair with finasteride, but this is the exception rather than the rule.

It's important to know that finasteride will only work as long as you're taking it. Within two to six months of discontinuing treatment with finasteride, the previous hair loss pattern will generally return to its state as if the medication had never been used.

Although many doctors will tell you that finasteride doesn't work for balding in the frontal area of the scalp, the FDA did approve it for this type of hair loss (see Chapter 18 for more on the FDA). Many people who have had early thinning in the frontal scalp may regrow hair if they start finasteride early in the thinning process. DHT causes frontal hair loss, and finasteride blocks the DHT impact on the loss of hair, but if there's no hair in the fontal area at all, you shouldn't expect any to appear.

You must take finasteride for at least one full year before your doctor can accurately determine its effects. During the first six months, you may note some thinning of existing hair as the new growing hair replaces the sickly miniaturized hair, so it's important to be patient during this period.

Does finasteride work for women?

There's some controversy on whether finasteride is effective in women. One study evaluating the efficacy of finasteride in post-menopausal women was terminated after one year with no significant hair growth.

Another study evaluated the effectiveness of the combination of a higher dose of oral finasteride (2.5 mg) with an oral contraceptive. This study only included perimenopausal women with pattern hair loss. After one year, 62 percent of the women in this study demonstrated some decrease of hair loss.

It's not clear if the success was due to the dosage (2.5 mg instead of 1 mg used in the previous study); the combination of use with an oral contraceptive containing drospirenone, which also has an effect on hair loss; or the fact that this study looked at peri-menopausal instead of postmenopausal females. The study group was too small to determine safety from a statistical point of view.

Finasteride has *not* been approved for women. In addition, women shouldn't handle crushed or broken Propecia tablets when they're pregnant or may potentially be pregnant because of the possibility of absorption through the skin and the subsequent potential risk to a male fetus in the first trimester of pregnancy. However, there appears to be no risk to the fetus if a man taking finasteride impregnates a woman.

As of this writing, finasteride isn't recommended for women to treat pattern hair loss. Further studies are needed to better understand which women may respond to treatment before its use can be advocated, and safety issues (including a possibility of increased risk of breast cancer) also need further investigation.

What are finasteride's side effects?

Side effects from Propecia at the standard 1 mg daily dose are rare, and fortunately if they do occur, they're not permanent.

In a study of men taking finasteride 1 mg, around 2 to 4 percent experienced some form of sexual dysfunction (decreased libido, erectile dysfunction, or decreased volume of ejaculate) compared to just over 2 percent of men treated with a placebo. For those men who reported cases of sexual dysfunction soon after starting the medication, it appeared generally within months. A small number of men saw a change in their libido or sexual function months or years into taking the drug.

You'll be happy to know that the sexual side effects were reversed in all men who discontinued therapy (and in 58 percent of those who continued treatment, the sexual side effects returned to their normal premedication levels). After the medication was stopped, all sexual side effects generally disappeared within a few weeks.

If you experience *negative* sexual side effects, you should consult with your doctor about stopping the medication until the side effects go away and then restarting at a lower dose (either a quarter or half of a 1 mg pill a day). If you have no side effects after several weeks on the lower dose, you can work back up to the 1 mg per day dose. Even staying on a lower dose will offer some benefit, but if side effects occur at the lower dose, it may be time to quit therapy with this medication.

Another rare side effect to be aware of is breast tenderness or breast enlargement (in males this is called *gynecomastia*). This occurred in 0.4 percent of men on finasteride 1 mg but was no greater than in the control group. In men who developed gynecomastia, the appearance of breast cancer was slightly higher than in the control group, although this connection may not be statistically significant.

Other side effects that were no more common than those experienced in patients taking a placebo included rash, itching, hives, swelling of the lips and face, and testicular pain. Some rare cases of mood changes have also been reported. There have been no interactions between finasteride 1 mg and any other drugs reported at the time of this writing.

Checking finasteride's effects on the prostate

Prostate specific antigen (PSA) levels are used to screen for prostate enlargement and prostate cancer. Finasteride causes a decrease in PSA blood levels by approximately 50 percent in healthy men; therefore, it's important that your doctor know if you're taking finasteride so that he or she may take this into account when interpreting your PSA results.

A study in 2003 on 5 mg finasteride reported that men treated with 5 mg finasteride for seven years had a 25 percent reduction in prostate cancer compared to men treated with placebo. The authors concluded that 5 mg finasteride prevents or delays the appearance of prostate cancer and that this possible benefit and a reduced risk of urinary problems must be weighed against sexual side effects and the remote possible increased risk of more aggressive prostate cancer.

Men aged 50 or over should inform their regular physicians or urologists if they're taking Finasteride 1 mg to treat hair loss. It's also recommended that all men aged 50 or over have routine annual evaluations for prostate disease, regardless of whether or not they're on Finasteride 1 mg. (African Americans or patients with a family history of prostate disease should start annuals exams at age 40.) An evaluation may include a rectal examination, a baseline PSA, and other tests that the physician feels are appropriate.

Proper dosing of finasteride

If your doctor prescribes finasteride to treat your hair loss, it's best to take the recommended dose of 1 mg per day as long as you have no side effects. Lower doses have been shown to be effective, but less so. There's also little evidence that a higher dose helps, although some doctors may increase the dose under certain circumstances. Studies don't yet show statistically valid connections between a higher dose of finasteride for the treatment of hair loss in men.

The 5 mg dose of finasteride now available in generic form is cheaper than five doses of Finasteride 1 mg. (The brand name of the 5 mg dose is Proscar.) You can use a pill cutter to divide the 5 mg tablet into approximately four pieces. Taking one piece every day is equivalent to 1.25 mg per day, but be advised that there's no scientific data ensuring that this is as effective as finasteride 1 mg.

Also, remember that there's a potential risk to pregnant women from handling broken or crushed tablets as finasteride can be absorbed through the skin.

Finasteride 1 mg isn't affected by food, so you can take it any time during the day without regard to meals. Taking it in the morning may have an advantage, though, because testosterone levels are highest in the morning in most men.

Combining finasteride and minoxidil

Finasteride and minoxidil (brand name Rogaine; see the section, "Stimulating Hair Growth with Minoxodil," later in this chapter) have an increased effect if taken together because they work differently. Finasteride permits hair growth by blocking the negative effects of DHT, whereas minoxidil stimulates the hair follicle directly. Of the two, finasteride is far more effective. There are no contradictions to taking the two together, and you may see better results by taking both regularly.

Dutasteride — Another Inhibitor of DHT

In 2002, the FDA approved a drug called Avodart (dutasteride 0.5 mg) for the treatment of prostate enlargement in men, but the drug also works to inhibit DHT and therefore permit hair growth. This section helps you understand dutasteride and how it may be able to treat your hair loss.

Dutasteride isn't approved specifically for the treatment of male pattern hair loss, and there are no long-term studies assessing its safety and efficacy in hair loss, although short-term study results have been promising.

How dutasteride works

Like finasteride, dutasteride inhibits the enzyme 5AR, which is responsible for the conversion of testosterone to DHT. However, unlike finasteride, which only inhibits one type of the enzyme, dutasteride inhibits both types, making the drug possibly more potent but also increasing the incidence of adverse reactions and side effects.

A dosage of dutasteride 0.5 mg per day decreases serum DHT 91 percent and scalp DHT 54 percent. In comparison, 5 mg finasteride decreases serum DHT 71 percent and scalp DHT 38 percent. Based on these numbers, you may expect dutasteride to be more effective in the treatment of male pattern hair loss than finasteride.

However, because the type of 5AR that dutasteride blocks isn't present in significant quantities in the hair follicle, the effects may not significant. Further studies are needed to answer this important question of which is more effective: dutasteride or finasteride.

Assessing the efficacy of dutasteride

Only a couple of studies have examined the effectiveness of dutasteride for pattern hair loss.

In 2007, a study was published that compared the efficacy of dutasteride to that of placebo in the treatment of androgenetic alopecia in 17 pairs of identical twin males over a one-year period. One twin from each pair received dutasteride 0.5 mg/day for 12 months while the other received placebo.

At the end of the study 15 of the 17 sets of twins correctly guessed which one was using dutasteride. The investigators concluded that dutasteride significantly improves hair growth and reduces hair loss progression in men with male pattern hair loss.

In 2006, a larger study was conducted with 416 men. The participants received either dutasteride (in doses of 0.05, 0.1, 0.5 or 2.5 mg), finasteride 5 mg, or placebo daily for 24 weeks. The investigators found that dutasteride increased area hair count versus placebo, with the level of success depending on the dosage.

In addition, dutasteride 2.5 mg was superior to finasteride 5 mg at 12 and 24 weeks. Scalp and serum dihydrotestosterone levels decreased, and testosterone levels increased, both with the level of success depending on the dosage. A major limitation of this study was that it was limited to only 24 weeks.

What are dutasteride's side effects?

Dutasteride has a greater incidence of sexual side effects compared to finasteride (refer to the earlier section "What are finasteride's side effects?"). Dutasteride was investigated in controlled multicenter studies involving men aged 50 and above with prostate enlargement. Drug-related side effects during the first six months included impotence (at 4.7 percent, the highest percentage of occurrence), decreased libido, ejaculation disorders, and breast tenderness and breast enlargement (at 0.5 percent, the lowest percentage of occurrence).

The good news is that most drug-related sexual side effects decreased with time in this study. However, drug-related breast tenderness and breast enlargement remained constant over the treatment period.

In recent cases, dutasteride has caused significant drops in sperm count, which could result in problems with male fertility.

As with finasteride, dutasteride reduces the amount of PSA measured in the blood, which must be taken into account when PSA levels are used in the detection of prostate cancer. Women who are pregnant or may become pregnant shouldn't handle dutasteride because of the possibility of absorbing it through the skin and subsequent potential risk to a male fetus.

Dutesteride hangs around in your bloodstream much longer that finasteride does; the half-life of dutasteride is five weeks compared to six to eight hours for finasteride, and blood tests can detect dutasteride in your system up to four to six months after you stop taking the drug. Therefore, you shouldn't donate blood until at least six months after you final dose of dutasteride to prevent giving it to a pregnant woman through a blood transfusion.

At the time of this writing, dutasteride is being researched in an approved FDA format. This study is expected to address all the issues concerning safety and effectiveness of dutasteride as well as the side effects mentioned in this chapter. Stay tuned and talk to your doctor.

Stimulating Hair Growth with Minoxidil

The first FDA-approved medication for the treatment of hair loss was topical minoxidil, also known by the brand name Rogaine. Rogaine is a topical solution that's applied directly to the scalp. Originally available only with a doctor's prescription, it's now available over-the-counter as both Rogaine and generic minoxidil solution, and it comes in concentrations of 5 percent for men and 2 percent for women. Recently, Rogaine developed a new minoxidil formulation in a 5 percent topical foam. This product is less greasy and easier to apply for some people.

How minoxidil works

Before minoxidil was available topically, it was an oral blood pressure medication. Doctors observed that many people taking oral minoxidil not only had a decrease in blood pressure but began growing body hair as well. It was reasoned that applying minoxidil directly to a bald scalp may cause hair to grow in this area without producing the side effects of the oral medication. Researchers developed a topical formulation, and studies showed modest hair growth on the scalp.

Just how minoxidil works in hair growth is unknown. The drug is a vasodilator (vasodilators cause the blood vessels to dilate, or expand) and may increase the flow of blood to the hair follicle, but how this relates to hair loss is unclear. In addition, minoxidil also increases the duration of the hair follicle growth cycle and improves the quality of the hair by increasing the diameter and length of fine, miniaturized hair.

How effective is minoxidil and on which areas of the scalp?

The original studies on minoxidil were performed on the crown of the head, so there's a misconception that it only works in this area. Although minoxidil may work best in the crown area, it also works to a lesser degree in other areas as long as there's some fine (miniaturized) hair (such as at the front of the scalp). However, it doesn't work if the area is totally bald.

The greatest benefit from minoxidil is visible between six months to two years from the beginning of treatment. After this time, you see a gradual decrease in effectiveness, so you'll continue to lose hair, but at a slower rate than if you weren't on the drug.

The effectiveness of minoxidil to treat men with pattern hair loss has been investigated since the mid-1980s and is well established. Even though both 5 percent and 2 percent solutions have been shown to decrease hair loss and increase hair, the 5 percent solution seems to work better.

If you stop using minoxidil, the effects wear off within three months, and the previous pattern of hair loss resumes. When you restart it, you generally don't regain the hair that was lost, so it's best not to stop and start the mediation but rather to use it regularly.

Does minoxidil work for women?

Yes, minoxidil works for women with pattern hair loss, but only the 2 percent concentration of minoxidil has been approved for their use. In 1994, a study was conducted in which 256 women with androgenic alopecia used 2 percent minoxidil twice daily for 32 weeks. At the end of the study, the investigators found that 60 percent of the patients in the 2 percent minoxidil group reported new hair growth compared with 40 percent of the patients in the placebo group.

The investigators concluded that minoxidil is an effective treatment for pattern hair loss in women but that it doesn't work on all patients.

Although the 2 percent minoxidil solution is the only approved dose in women, there's evidence that the 5 percent solution may be superior. In 2004, a study with 381 female patients with pattern hair loss was conducted comparing 5 percent minoxidil with 2 percent minoxidil. Both strengths were shown to help regrow hair, but the 5 percent topical minoxidil group demonstrated superiority over the 2 percent group.

What are minoxodil's side effects?

By far the most common side effect of topical minoxidil is local irritation, although the foam formulation is much less irritating than the original version.

Another side effect sometimes seen in women is the development of facial hair. Although this may decrease when the medication is discontinued, at times the hair may need to be removed after treatment with either electrolysis or lasers. To reduce the chances of this problem (although you can't eliminate it entirely), you should be careful when applying minoxidil and try to avoid the medication dripping down onto the temples and forehead, unless, of course, a hairy forehead is the look you're going for! (Although the 2 percent solution is standard for women, there's a significantly greater incidence of this side effect when the 5 percent solution is used.)

Female patients also seem to be more sensitive to the potential systemic side effects of minoxidil in decreasing blood pressure (a condition called *hypotension*). Rarely women may get lightheaded (a symptom of low blood pressure) from topically applying minoxidil. Women also have an increased risk of developing allergic skin reactions on the scalp.

It is important to know that minoxidil can cause birth defects. Women who are pregnant, planning to become pregnant, or nursing shouldn't use this medication.

Comparing minoxidil to finasteride

Studies have demonstrated that minoxidil is an inferior treatment for male pattern hair loss compared to finasteride. In 2004, a study was conducted in which male androgenetic alopecia patients used either 1 mg oral finasteride or 5 percent topical minoxidil twice daily for one year. Eighty percent of the men using finasteride and 52 percent of those using minoxidil had an increase in hair density. The study demonstrated that while both medications are effective, finasteride is superior. Additional studies have shown that the combination of finasteride with minoxidil is superior to finasteride alone, which suggests a synergistic effect, meaning that two medications together work better than either medication used alone.

Applying minoxidil

Doctors recommend that you apply minoxidil directly to the scalp (not the hair) twice a day. In order to regain lost hair, you need to apply the solution to all thinning areas, including the frontal hairline and temples.

Once a day topical use of minoxidil is probably almost as effective as twice a day use because it has a long half-life of almost 24 hours. Once a day dosing is a reasonable option if it's not practical for you to apply it twice daily.

In fact, a study in 2007 showed that using a combination of 5 percent minoxidil and 0.01 percent tretinoin (a cream that makes the minoxidil penetrate the scalp better) once a day was equivalent conventional 5 percent minoxidil twice-daily therapy for the treatment of pattern hair loss in men.

One caveat is that topical tretinoin can sometimes be irritating to the scalp and may increase the amount of minoxidil entering the bloodstream, which could result in unwanted side effects (covered in the earlier section, "What are minoxidil's side effects?").

Medications for Women Only

Two prescription medications for women with pattern hair loss deserve special mention: spironolactone and cyproterone acetate. Both are *anti-androgens,* meaning they suppress the actions of testosterone, and have been studied in women to treat female pattern hair loss. These medications should be used by women only; for men, they cause decreased sex drive and other unacceptable side effects.

Spironolactone

Spironolactone (brand name Aldactone) is an oral diuretic (or *water pill*) that's FDA-approved to treat congestive heart failure and high blood pressure. The drug also has been shown in a few small studies to help reduce unwanted hair in females and has been studied in women with pattern hair loss — but with mixed results. It may have some effect in reducing thinning in women with very limited pattern hair loss.

Spironolactone has been associated with an increased risk of bleeding from the gastrointestinal tract, although a definite link hasn't been established. It isn't used in men because it can cause testicular atrophy and breast enlargement as well as decreased sexual function.

Cyproterone acetate

Because it's an anti-androgen (anti-androgens block the effects of male hormones in women), cyproterone acetate should be used only by women. A few studies have been published documenting mild effectiveness of cyproterone acetate in the treatment of both hirsutism (excessive hairiness) and female pattern hair loss. It's available in combination with estrogen for use as an oral contraceptive in Europe, but it's not FDA-approved and not available in the U.S.

The most serious potential side effect of cyproterone acetate is liver toxicity; the drug also has been linked to increased rate of blood clots.

Chapter 10

Supplementing Your Diet to Help Slow Hair Loss

. . . .

In This Chapter

▶ Eating healthy to preserve and protect your hair

▶ Exploring alternative hair loss treatments: Oils and herbs

▶ Staying informed about unproven hair loss treatment ingredients

. . . .

*E*verything in your body — including your hair — maintains its
health and vitality thanks to what you put into it. Can you
avoid baldness forever by consuming enough protein, vitamins,
and minerals? Probably not (forever is a tall order, after all), but
you may be able to slow or avoid hair loss caused by nutritional
deficiencies — and you can keep the hair you have looking healthy
and at its best.

In this chapter, we start with the big picture of how diet and nutrition affect hair. Then we explain the affects of various vitamins and
minerals and look at ancient remedies for hair loss and the treatments still used today in traditional Chinese and Indian medicine.

Although there hasn't been a great deal of scientific research into
whether herbs and oils delay or prevent hair loss, the treatments
we describe have been used for many years in alternative medicine. We also warn you about treatments that don't work — and
that could be harmful to your health.

Eating Your Way to Healthy Hair

Everybody knows that eating well is essential for a healthy heart,
bones, and other key body systems, but you may not realize that a
lack of protein, good fat, vitamins, and minerals can affect what
grows out of the top of your head as well. Hair needs to be fed —
and fed well — to keep growing and to stay put. A steady diet of
junk food isn't healthy fodder for your hair.

People who don't eat meat or dairy products may be missing out on important vitamins and minerals necessary for hair health.

Pumping up calories and proteins

It's well documented that a diet deficient in calories or protein can contribute to hair loss or hair that doesn't look healthy and vibrant. For example, patients with anorexia nervosa, a disease in which the patient consumes too few calories to sustain good health, often experience hair loss. Hair without good luster doesn't feel good when you run your fingers through it, or it may be brittle and break off easily — all may reflect a nutritional problem with your diet.

You can get most of the amino acids your body needs from a proper, well-balanced diet, but others are harder to absorb from the diet, especially as you get older. For some people, protein supplements may have a beneficial affect on hair growth.

Adequate protein intake is critical for hair growth including amino acids, which include lysine, arginine, cystine, cysteine, and methionine. These amino acids are created by the body from the proteins we eat. If you eat protein rich foods, you get enough of these essential amino acids, but if you don't, supplements may provide some of them. The essential amino acids are found in lean meats, nuts, grains, soy, fish, eggs, and dairy products.

Two sulfur-containing amino acids, methionine and cysteine, are most important for maintaining hair health because human hair requires sulfur for normal growth. (The body also requires sulfur for healthy connective tissue formation.)

- **Methionine:** Methionine is an essential amino acid that your body doesn't produce, so it must come from your diet or from supplements. Foods rich in methionine include sesame seeds, fish, meats, and some other plant seeds.

  The current recommended dose of methionine is 250 milligrams per day. Taking too much of this amino acid can cause toxicity because methionine is broken down into homocysteine, which can lead to heart disease.

- **Cysteine:** Cysteine supports hair growth by providing sulfur to replicating hair follicle cells. It's a non-essential amino acid, which means that your body can make it on its own. Cysteine also is found in most high-protein foods, including eggs, milk, whey protein, some cheese, chicken, turkey, and duck. Vegetarian sources include red peppers, garlic, brussel sprouts, oats, and wheat.

The recommended dose of cysteine is 100 milligrams per day. Supplementing your diet with cysteine has the affect of increasing the sulfur percentage in hair, which has been reported to increase the thickness and the strength of the hair.

Fitting in the good fats

"Good fats," or essential fatty acids such as omega-3 and omega-6 oils, are essential for your body's functioning but are only obtained through your diet — your body can't manufacture these. You can get these essential fatty acids from fish (salmon, sardines, tuna), plant (flaxseed, soybeans, pumpkin seeds), and nut (walnut) oils, as well as in fish oil capsules.

After two to four months of essential fatty acid deficiency, people report hair dryness, change of hair color, scalp redness, and flakes. Consuming unsaturated fatty acids, for example fish oil or evening primrose oil, has been found to improve hair texture and scalp redness after a few months.

On the other hand, some people believe that a diet too heavy in saturated animal fat may contribute to hair loss. Evidence comes from the effects of dietary change seen in Japanese men. After World War II, more Japanese men started consuming greater amounts of saturated animal fats, and they also started complaining of hair loss. Although this interesting relationship doesn't prove cause and effect, it does show one possible effect of diet on your hair.

In traditional Indian medicine, body weakness is believed to cause hair loss, and so one treatment consists of a diet rich in proteins, including meat, fish (source of essential fatty acids), and dairy products. Avoidance of fried foods (source of saturated fats) is also recommended.

Getting your daily vitamins

Vitamins are organic compounds necessary to sustain life. You need to get your vitamins from food or dietary supplements, because you can't make them yourself. Most vitamins work to speed up critical chemical reactions in the body.

Vitamins are important nutrients for healthy hair. Don't start taking vitamins by the handful to make sure you're getting your daily requirement, though; doctors have linked hair loss to both deficiencies of some vitamins and excesses of others, and some vitamins can be dangerous to your overall health if you take too many.

The following sections run through the vitamins you need and the quantities that are helpful for your hair — and the rest of you!

Vitamin A

Vitamin A protects hair follicles from damage by free radicals, which are atoms with an unpaired electron. A diet deficient in vitamin A is also known to cause dry hair.

Too much vitamin A has been linked to hair loss. Vitamin A is a fat-soluble vitamin, which means that excess amounts are stored in the body and not washed out in urine, so it's essential to keep vitamin A intake within normal limits.

Foods high in vitamin A include carrots, broccoli, and liver. The current recommendation of daily vitamin A intake is 900 micrograms (mcg) (3,000 IU) for men and 700 micrograms (2,300 IU) for women.

B-complex vitamins

The B vitamins include thiamin, riboflavin, niacin, pyridoxine, cobalmin, and pantothenic acid. B vitamins are believed to contribute to the nourishment of the hair follicle.

You can get B vitamins from foods such as potatoes, bananas, tuna, and turkey. Deficiency in B vitamins has been associated with anemia and neurologic problems.

- **Biotin:** Also known as vitamin H or B7, biotin is a water-soluble B-complex vitamin that's required for cell growth, the production of fatty acids, and the metabolism of amino acids. An adequate amount of biotin is about 30 to 100 mcg daily. Biotin is found in many foods including beans, bread, fish, and legumes.

  Biotin deficiency has been strongly linked to hair loss and, when severe, can even lead to loss of the eyebrows and lashes. Deficiency is rare but can be caused by excessive consumption of raw eggs, which contain high levels of the protein avidin, which strongly binds biotin.

- **Folic acid:** This is the synthesized form of folate, which is important to maintain hair follicle cell division and growth. Rich sources of folate include leafy vegetables such as spinach, lettuce, dried beans, and other fruits and vegetables. The current recommendation for folate intake is 400 mcg per day. However, if you're pregnant or nursing, you should ask your doctor for a recommended dosage.

Signs of folic acid deficiency include anemia, increased fatigue, sore tongue, and graying hair. There's evidence that exposure to ultraviolet light, including the use of tanning beds, can lead to a folic acid deficiency. In addition certain medicines, such as methotrexate used to treat severe psoriasis and some forms of cancer, can lead to deficiency.

Vitamin C

Vitamin C is required to maintain healthy collagen in the connective tissue in your body and also around hair follicles. It also protects your cells because it's a strong antioxidant (a substance that reduces damage caused by free radicals, which contribute to aging changes and can cause problems in many body systems).

Citrus fruit is a rich source of vitamin C. Currently, the recommended dose of vitamin C is 90 milligrams per day and no more than 2 grams per day.

The most famous condition associated with vitamin C deficiency is scurvy, which results when collagen stops functioning properly. Symptoms of scurvy include bleeding gums, nose bleeds, sunken eyes, dark purplish spots on the legs, pinpoint bleeding around hair follicles, as well as unique "corkscrew hairs." Fortunately, this disease is rare in industrialized countries where fruits and vegetables are plentiful in the diet.

Vitamin E

Vitamin E is the collective name for a set of eight related fat-soluble vitamins with antioxidant properties. Vitamin E provides physical stability to cell membranes, including cell membranes of hair follicles. Nuts, corn, and asparagus are just a few foods with high vitamin E levels. The daily recommendation of vitamin E for adults is 8 to 10 mg.

Vitamin E deficiency is rare and usually manifests first with neurologic deterioration, such as loss of reflexes.

A recent study from Johns Hopkins University showed that taking vitamin E supplements in amounts greater than 400 IU a day may actually be harmful to your health, increasing your risk of death from a number of causes.

IU is dependent on the potency of the substance, and each substance would have a different IU to milligram conversion. For example, 1,000 IU of Vitamin C would have a different weight than 1,000 IU of Vitamin A. Because each substance would have a different conversion ratio, we cannot state a conversion for IU to milligrams that covers everything, or even most things. There are just too many different substances.

The Helsinki Formula failure

In the 1980s, niacin was combined with polysorbate 80 and vitamin B6 and marketed under the name Helsinki Formula. Heavy promotion led to the first large market for a hair-loss product. The concoction proved to be ineffective, though, and the Helsinki Formula lost its $100 million market. But its marketing efforts opened eyes to a marketing field ripe with people willing to try anything to keep or replace their hair, which has spurred the development of hundreds of hair loss products and a billion-dollar business in the 21st century.

Minding your mineral intake

Minerals are inorganic elements that are essential to the functioning of the human body and are obtained from foods. Minerals necessary to maintain hair health include copper, iodine, iron, selenium, silica, and zinc. Table 10-1 lays them all out for you.

Table 10-1   Minerals Important for Healthy Hair

Mineral	What It Does	Results of Deficiency	Recommended Daily Intake for Adults	Sources
Copper	Essential for proper enzyme function in all plants and animals	Associated with hair loss, anemia, diarrhea, and weakness	0.9 mg For pregnant women 1mg, for lactating women 1.3 mgs. For everyone else 0.9 mgs	Seafood such as oysters, squid, lobster, nuts almonds and pistachios, egumes (soy beans, lentils, chocolate)
Iodine	Keeps the thyroid gland functioning (see Chapter 6)	Can lead to hypothyroidism, which causes weight gain, lethargy, change in hair texture, and hair loss	150 mcg for both men and women	Some seafood and plants, and iodized salt

Mineral	What It Does	Results of Deficiency	Recommended Daily Intake for Adults	Sources
Iron	Is incorporated into an essential component of hemoglobin, which transports oxygen through the body	Causes anemia, brittle hair, and hair loss	Varies by age gender, and dietary source; excessive amounts may be problematic and lead to liver damage; ask your doctor	Red meat, fish, poultry, and leafy vegetables
Selenium	Required for proper functioning of the thyroid gland (see Chapter 6)	Associated with heart disease and poor hair growth	55 mcg for both men and women	Nuts, meat, fish, crab, lobster, and eggs
Silica	Used in the formation of keratin sulfate, a component of the hair shaft; also may increase scalp circulation and stimulate hair growth	Weakening of bones and teeth, hardening of the arteries	There is no recommended daily dose but doses of greater than 20 micrograms per day is dangerous	Sand, opal, and agate; also in horsetail extract, barley, hile grains, leafy green vegetables, rice
Zinc	Required in DNA replication and RNA production and necessary to maintain normal hair follicle cell division	Effects of deficiency; typically the result of inadequate zinc in the diet (common in people who don't eat meat)	11 mg for men; 8 mg for women (higher amounts recommended during pregnancy and lactation)	Oysters, animal proteins, beans, nuts, grains, and various seeds

Oils, Herbs, and Extracts: Alternative Hair Loss Remedies

Concern over hair loss has plagued men and women for thousands of years, and hair loss remedies go back almost as far. The ancient Egyptians applied concoctions directly to the scalp or consumed them to try to combat the balding process. The famous Greek physician Hippocrates is rumored to have applied pigeon droppings to his scalp in hopes to regrow hair. And in colonial times, America's balding forefathers donned white wigs to cover shiny scalps. There has been no lack of creative cover-ups or attempts to save rapidly receding hairlines over the years.

Here, we review some alternative, but not scientifically proven, methods of keeping hair where it belongs, including ancient Chinese and Indian oils and herbs.

Oiling it up

Oiling your hair may seem a little out of date, but over the years, many people have used oils to stimulate hair growth. For example, the ancient Egyptians were very concerned about maintaining thick hair and believed that castor oil applied to the scalp could stimulate hair growth. (They sometimes mixed it with sweet almond oil to improve the smell.) Ancient Indians and Polynesians used coconut oil, and ancient Africans used olive oil, all applied to the hair and scalp in an attempt to stimulate hair growth.

At least one current study shows that oil application can help with some specific types of hair loss. In 1998, researchers from Scotland published their results of a randomized, double-blind controlled study investigating aromatherapy in patients with alopecia areata, a condition in which the body's immune cells start attacking healthy hair-producing cells. (We cover it in Chapter 5.)

In this study, 86 patients were placed into two different groups. One (the active group) massaged their scalps daily with four essential oils (thyme, rosemary, lavender, and cedar wood) in a mixture of jojoba and grape seed oils. The other group (the control group) massaged only jojoba and grape seed oils into their scalps daily. Each group massaged the oils into their scalps for a total of seven months.

Interestingly, 19 of 43 patients (44 percent) in the active group showed improvement compared with only 6 of 41 patients (15 percent) in the control group. The authors concluded that aromatherapy with these essential oils may be a safe and effective treatment for alopecia areata.

Helping hair with herbs

In recent years, growing concern about potential short- and long-term side effects of pharmaceuticals and conventional medical treatments have led to an increase in popularity of alternative medicines and herbal therapies. This trend affects all aspects of medicine, including increased interest in seeking herbal remedies for hair loss.

It's important to remember that "natural" doesn't always mean "harmless." Also, there's no way to be sure exactly how much herbal remedy is in a purchased product. Herbal products supposedly containing the same amount of medication have been found to vary considerably under testing.

Herbals aren't like FDA-approved medicines, and few herbal remedies have been studied in a controlled fashion for hair loss. Many are advertised as miracle treatments with little evidence to support the claims that they're either safe or effective. This doesn't mean that they don't work to regrow hair, just that there's not enough scientific evidence to support that claim.

The bottom line is this: Before you decide to ingest or topically apply something to any part of your body, including your head, don't assume that product is safe just because it's labeled "natural." The following sections get into a number of alternative medicines. Our goal in sharing this information isn't to advocate the use, or disuse, of these products but merely to present them in as scientific a manner as possible.

Saw palmetto

Saw palmetto is a small plum plant endemic to the southeastern United States. It's believed that the medicinal properties of the plant come from its brown-black berries.

Native Americans used saw palmetto to relieve urinary symptoms in older men who had difficulty urinating. Over the years, several studies have documented the effectiveness of saw palmetto in the treatment of benign prostate gland enlargement (BPH), and it's used quite frequently in Europe.

Saw palmetto has also gained popularity as an herbal remedy for androgenic alopecia, or male pattern baldness, although there's far less scientific evidence that it works to prevent hair loss.

Although the exact mechanism isn't fully understood, several basic research studies have demonstrated that saw palmetto blocks the enzyme *5-alpha-reductase,* which functions to convert testosterone to DHT, the male hormone responsible for male pattern baldness (see Chapter 4 for more about DHT).

Only one study examining saw palmetto to treat male pattern baldness has been published in the medical literature. In this small study, six out of ten subjects with androgenic alopecia who received saw palmetto benefited from the treatment. This is far too small a study to draw any conclusions on whether saw palmetto actually works to treat pattern hair loss.

 Saw palmetto has several potential side effects. The most common are mild and include abdominal pain, diarrhea, nausea and vomiting, and constipation. Men taking saw palmetto have also reported erectile dysfunction, breast tenderness or enlargement, and loss of libido.

 If you're taking hormone medications for hair loss, such as Propecia, you shouldn't take saw palmetto because combining these two may increase the way your body reacts to them. You also shouldn't take saw palmetto without medical supervision if you're on blood thinners, and the use of saw palmetto by pregnant or nursing women should be avoided as there has been no safety testing in this population.

Traditional Chinese medicine

Pattern baldness is relatively less common among the Asian population than among Caucasians; many believe this may be related to diet, although the Asian hair type and heredity may also play a part. Asians have a diet rich in vegetables and herbs, some of which may help fight hair loss.

Researchers have found that a series of amino acids found in legumes and vegetables inhibit the enzyme 5-alpha-reductase Type II, which converts testosterone to DHT, the male hormone responsible for male pattern baldness (see Chapter 4). Excess amounts of zinc taken in supplements can have the same effect. If these reports are accurate and reproducible, then the use of certain amino acids and zinc may slow down hair loss, much like the use of certain drugs such as finasteride and dutasteride.

 Roasted sesame seeds are an herbal food used for hundreds of years in Chinese medicine. They're believed to decrease hair loss and possibly stimulate hair regrowth.

The following sections take a close look at two Chinese herbal remedies with long histories.

He Shou Wu

Many believe that the Chinese herb *He Shou Wu,* also known as *Polygoni multiflori* or *Fo Ti,* stimulates hair growth and also converts fine vellus hair to thicker terminal hair. It may also delay natural graying. Practitioners of Chinese medicine use He Shou Wu for other conditions, such as strengthening weak bones, decreasing high blood pressure, and treating constipation. It's also thought to have anti-aging properties.

To obtain a benefit from He Shou Wu, you have to ingest the root powder for several months. Known side effects include headaches and diarrhea.

Recently, the Medicines and Health Care Products Regulatory Agency (MHRA) in London released a warning about potential liver damage from the use of He Shou Wu. The MHRA advises that anyone with elevated liver enzymes or liver disease avoid this product until they discuss it with their doctor.

In 2002, a controlled clinical trial was conducted using a combination of oral tablets and lotion containing He Shou Wu. While the final groups were of very small sample size, results did favor the group who received the active herbal ingredients. However, you can't draw any definitive conclusions from such a small study, and further research is needed to confirm the results.

Dabao

In 1991, researchers from the Netherlands studied the effectiveness of the Chinese herb extract *Dabao* for the treatment of male pattern baldness. In this study, 373 people with androgenic alopecia completed the full six-month trial. At the end of the study, the authors concluded that over a six-month period, Dabao has a (albeit modest) cosmetic effect superior to placebo.

Ayurvedic remedies

Ayurvedic medicine is an alternative medical practice based on the traditional medicine of India. The word *Ayurveda* is derived from a combination of two Sanskrit terms: *ayu* meaning "life," and *veda* meaning "knowledge" or "science." The practice of Ayurvedic medicine is believed to be over 5,000 years old in India, and it uses a number of herbs to help prevent hair loss, including

- ✔ *Bhringaraj (Eclipta alba)*, which is believed to promote new hair growth and also bring back natural hair color in people who are graying.

- ✔ *Gotu kola (Centella asiatica)*, very commonly used to treat hair loss as well as to stimulate brain cells, being believed to help with memory and longevity.

- ✔ *Tridax procumbens, amalaki, sandalwood (Santalum)*, and *licorice (Hlycyrrhiza glabra)*, all of which may stimulate hair growth.

In 2007 researchers in India tested the combination of extracts from three traditional Indian herbs to see what affects they would have on hair growth in rats. The topical formulation sped up hair growth on shaved rats, and analysis of the hair growth cycle after treatment revealed more hair follicles in the anagen phase, when hair cells grow rapidly, compared with controls.

Additional herbal remedies

- ✔ **Herbal tea:** To treat hair loss, brew an herbal tea with a combination of nettle tea, sage, and rosemary. No time for a cup of tea? Apply the mixture directly to your scalp! (No, we're not kidding.) No matter how you use it, herbal tea is thought to cause hair growth by improving blood flow to the scalp.

- ✔ **Procyanidin B-2:** This extract from apples has been shown to promote hair growth in a laboratory study. Perhaps the old adage "An apple a day keeps the doctor away" may soon change to "An apple a day keeps the hair loss away!"

- ✔ **Procyanidolic oligomers (PCOs):** Extracts from the French maritime pine bark and grape seeds belong to this family of antioxidant substances. One POC may have the effects of stimulating hair growth, but more studies are needed to confirm this.

- ✔ **Horsetail extract:** This herb is a natural source of cysteine, selenium, and silica, which we discuss in the sections "Pumping up calories and proteins" and Table 10-1, earlier in this chapter.

Potions, Mixtures, and Other Dubious Products

We try to protect our patients from the unknown. When we don't know something to be proven, we remind ourselves of how many undocumented side effects or enzyme defects occur that are caused by natural herbs that could threaten a person's health or life because they're not researched or understood. For example, arsenic is a natural substance used historically to treat syphilis, but we wouldn't recommend arsenic as an alternative to modern antibiotics, which are safe, well tested, FDA regulated, and accepted worldwide.

The supplements and substances listed in this section may not be covered in the FDA regulatory process that confirms dosages, purity, safety, and efficacy. The research and studies that show efficacy are often funded by the supplement manufacturers, which obviously may bias the reported results. Finally, the proper dosages for such products seem arbitrary and unproven. Just because the friendly neighborhood natural food outlet sales staff are dressed in white lab coats and attest to the efficacy of a homeopathic product doesn't mean that these are safe and/or effective.

This exhausting — but not exhaustive — list of herbals, minerals, vegetables, and combinations of these substances may be packaged into products that make claims for hair regrowth:

- **Advecia:** Herbal reported to be a hair loss vitamin.

- **Aloe vera:** Plant extract with many uses reported in topical use. The leaf of the plant exudes a white, sticky substance that has been claimed to be a strong topical agent used for medicinal purposes.

- **Dehydroepiandrosterone (DHEA):** Although suggested for hair growth, there are many reports that this hormone actually causes hair loss, possibly working in a way similar to steroids.

- **Evening promise oil:** Capsules contain gamma-linolenic acid, which is claimed to convert into hormone-like compounds that help regulate a number of bodily functions.

- **Fava beans:** Fava is an herb widely used in Polynesia to treat anxiety. Though harmless, fava beans can cause death in very small quantities in people who carry a rare genetic defect.

- **L-Arginine:** Homeopathic remedy thought to increase circulation to the scalp.

- **Lingzhi:** Flat polypore mushroom used to treat hair loss, obesity, and liver disease in traditional Chinese medicine.

- **Methylsulfonylmethane (MSM):** White, crystalline powder that's odorless and nearly tasteless. It's reported to be a sulphur-rich hair tonic in its cream form, but it's also known to be quite smelly!

✔ **Nettle sting root:** Reported effect on dihydrotestosterone (DHT) levels has also made it a treatment for hair loss.

✔ **Olive oil:** Claims abound that it can grow hair, particularly when mixed with coconut oil and/or mayonnaise, heated, and rubbed into the scalp.

✔ **Soy extract:** May arrest hair loss.

✔ **Tribulus terrestri and Ava Renewale:** Reported natural Chinese herbs that seem to do everything and anything; they're proposed as a cure for many conditions, including hair loss.

✔ **Wheatgrass:** Young version of the common wheat plant that can be a source of vitamins A, B, C, and E; as well as calcium, magnesium, potassium, iron, natural enzymes, and chlorophyll.

The following items are manufactured products that may include the ingredients in the previous list:

✔ **Ervamatin:** Hair lotion composed of herbs and plants from the Amazon rain forest.

✔ **Eucapil:** Approved as a cosmetic hair care agent for topical use in the Czech and Slovak Republics.

✔ **Hairgenesis:** Botanical that has claims of blocking DHT, a labeling violation under FDA labeling rules.

✔ **Himalaya Hair Loss Cream:** An Ayurvedic preparation (refer to the earlier section "Ayurvedic remedies").

✔ **Nutrifolica:** Manufacturer claims this 100 percent pure herbal extract is designed to counteract hair loss causes such as poor scalp circulation, clogged hair follicles, and excessive sebaceous oil.

✔ **NutriSol-RM, or Scalp Med:** Proprietary formulation packaged with essential amino acids and other agents. It claims to ensure optimal delivery of growth agents and nutrients to the matrix cells in the bulb of hair to revitalize the follicle, helping to grow hair.

✔ **Procerin:** Invalid claim to be a vitamin for hair loss that's specially formulated to block production of DHT, the primary cause of hair loss in men.

✔ **Provillis:** Nutritional supplement claimed to contain all-natural herbal ingredients that aren't specified.

✔ **Shen Min:** Chinese medicinal line of natural dietary supplements designed to help reduce hair loss and enhance hair growth in men and women. It's a combination of "standard-ized" herbs such as He Shou Wu and horse chestnut extract with nutrients such as silica and biotin.

✔ **T Bomb 2:** Product that claims to block estrogen and enhance testosterone and contains many and varied ingredients, making it potentially dangerous.

Chapter 11

Low-Level Laser Therapy

*W*hen people hear the words "laser" and "hair" in the same sentence, they usually think of hair removal. Although lasers work for hair removal, they may possibly also stimulate hair growth if used properly, although there haven't been enough scientific studies to prove this beyond any doubt.

In this chapter, we look at the role of lasers in hair replacement, the pros and cons of using lasers, and the results you can reasonably expect from laser treatment, as well as potential problems associated with lasers and the question of whether they really work for most people.

Discovering Lasers

The term *laser* is an acronym that stands for "light amplification by the stimulated emission of radiation." Credit for the initial theory behind lasers goes to Albert Einstein, but many other scientists took his lead and further advanced this technology.

Lasers sound high tech and complicated, and they are, but they're easier to understand than you may think. In the next sections, we discuss how lasers were invented, what they can do, and the differences in high-power and low-power laser therapy.

How laser therapy works

You've all seen lasers used in movies to defeat the evil empire, but lasers are no longer just part of science fiction. Lasers, which are thin, intensely focused light beams which emit a very pure light of one wavelength, have many medical applications today, and are being touted as a possible stimulus for hair growth in balding areas.

Most lasers used for cosmetic purposes target specific *chromophores* (components in the skin that absorb light) in the body. The major chromophores that affect your hair are

- ✔ **Melanin** (in hair follicles and sun spots)
- ✔ **Hemoglobin** (in blood vessels)
- ✔ **Water** (throughout the *epidermis* and *dermis* — layers of your skin)

Medical lasers can be either high or low powered. There's no question that high powered lasers are very effective in treating a number of medical conditions.

High-powered lasers are used to destroy hair follicles and remove unwanted hair, target abnormal blood vessels (such as varicose veins), and erase fine lines and wrinkles. High powered lasers can cut through tissue, burn tissue, and emit heat.

Low-level lasers, on the other hand, don't produce heat, and are generally used to heal damaged tissue rather than to destroy tissue.

Low-level laser therapy (LLLT) may stimulate better hair growth in an area that still has hair; it's not effective in growing new hair in a completely bald area.

Low-level laser therapy

Low-level laser therapy is a non-invasive technology that has been around for many years. Its main uses have been to stimulate wound healing, decrease inflammation, and lessen intense chronic pain.

The first low-level therapeutic laser was developed in the 1960s by Hungary's Endre Mester. He reported an improved healing of wounds through low-level laser treatment.

When used for hair loss, the theory is that chromophores absorb the laser light, which then stimulates hair growth in balding areas, possibly by increasing blood flow and increased oxygen flow to the area, which may stimulate the hair follicle at the cellular level and cause weak or thin hair to become stronger and thicker. We say "possibly" because this theory has yet to be scientifically proven.

Some clinicians believe these effects are due to a photochemical reaction produced by the interaction of the laser light with the hair follicle. This reaction alters the cell's internal processing and signals it to start growing rather than slowly dying.

Hairs that have already begun to *miniaturize* (thin in diameter) apparently respond to treatment, though completely bald areas typically do not respond. It takes typically up to 12 months to see any new hair growth, if it happens at all.

Who benefits from LLLT?

Both men and women experiencing *androgenic alopecia,* or genetic induced pattern baldness, appear to be the best candidates for LLLT. Some evidence suggests that LLLT works better when used in conjunction with minoxidil (topical over the counter medication for hair growth) and/or finasteride (prescription pill). (See Chapter 9 for more on both medications.)

Because LLLT isn't particularly effective on bald areas, it may be a more effective treatment in women, whose hair loss is typically *diffuse* (spread throughout the scalp) and more miniaturized, than in men, who typically have more areas of the scalp that are totally bald.

Note that laser therapy does not lead to permanent results. You must continue therapy in order for the hair to keep growing.

Looking at the clinical data

The clinical data for LLLT relating to hair loss isn't as plentiful as it is for proven treatments such as minoxidil and finasteride (see Chapter 9 for more on these medications). Although numerous reports and studies document its effectiveness, none of these studies were conducted in a controlled manner over a long period of time (greater than six months). Many reports of success with LLLT are anecdotal from individuals.

This lack of evidence does not mean that it doesn't work, but it does underscore the need for in-depth, long-term studies on the effectiveness of LLLT.

In 2003, a peer-reviewed medical journal published the first study looking at the effectiveness of a handheld LLLT device for the treatment of hair loss. Thirty-five patients diagnosed with androgenic alopecia participated in this study (28 male, 7 female); each got the handheld device for use at home for five to ten minutes every other day for six months.

After six months of use, hair counts in the temples increased by an average of 55 percent in females and 74 percent in males. In the *vertex* (crown of the scalp), the increase was 65 percent for females and 120 percent for men.

In total, for both areas, hair count increased by an average of 94 percent. In addition, the study reported an increase in hair strength.

Although these numbers sound very positive, put them in perspective. For example, one male patient had a total of 12 hairs in the counted area at baseline and then 23 hairs six months later. This change corresponded to an increase in hairs of 92 percent. In reality, though, 11 extra hairs probably didn't make a huge difference in his physical appearance, and the data was highly suspect when analyzed by these authors.

Finding a Physician

We recommend that you contact a physician who has experience in diagnosing the cause of hair loss before beginning LLLT therapy either in the doctor's office or at home, because other equally or more-effective treatments may be available to you; you may also be able to use these other treatments in conjunction with LLLT to enhance your results.

Combined therapy makes sense, as you may get complementary benefits from the different approaches, and one type of therapy may enhance the other.

Dermatologists are specifically trained in the diagnosis and treatment of hair loss, so consider starting with them. Check out www.aad.org for a list of dermatologists. Head to www.ishrs.org to find doctors who specialize in the surgical treatment of hair loss and who also have knowledge of LLLT treatments.

LLLT systems available in the doctor's office involve the patient sitting under the machine, an experience similar to sitting under a hair dryer at the hair salon. The advantages of having laser done in the office include the following:

- ✔ The lasers are stronger.
- ✔ You get a precise amount of laser delivered each time.
- ✔ It's less stressful than trying to do it yourself.
- ✔ Results are better-monitored over time by a doctor.

The disadvantages of the office-based system are

- ✔ You have to leave home to have it done.
- ✔ You have to make multiple trips to the office.
- ✔ It's much more expensive than doing it yourself.

Treatments are generally administered two or three times per week for 6 weeks and then once a week for the next 16 weeks. After observable hair growth occurs, periodic touch-ups may be needed to maintain the benefits of the treatment. Each treatment session takes approximately 20 minutes.

The doctor's office based systems generally price the service for a three or six month course of therapy with up to three visits per week at a cost of a few thousand dollars.

As of this writing, the in-office systems have been issued an *accession number* by the FDA, meaning the products are classified as cosmetic products and have met the international laser standards for safety. However, they're not yet FDA cleared for hair growth because scientific proof is lacking.

Manufacturers of the devices claim that studies with this type of machine have shown an 85 percent success rate in halting the progression of hair loss and up to a 39 percent increase in fullness, but again, scientific studies are lacking to confirm this.

Office-based treatments come in two varieties: a system with fixed diodes and a system with moving diodes.

In the fixed or static system, approximately 100 diodes (an electrical device which has two wires leading into them to produce a flow of electricity, in one side and out the other), each emitting light at a wavelength of about 650mn, are set into an apparatus that sits over the person's head.

The moving-diode system utilizes Rotational Phototherapy (RPT), in which 30 laser diodes rotate 180 degrees around the scalp. This process supposedly increases the contact of the laser energy with the hair follicles around the entire scalp and is potentially more effective in stimulating hair growth than other types of lasers.

The "shade covering" caused by your hair may block the laser from reaching the scalp, but in the moving diode systems, a new position assures more laser penetration through the hair and into the scalp.

Doing It Yourself: Hand-held Home-use Lasers

You may be interested in trying out an LLLT device, but aren't willing to put out the time and effort, not to mention the cash, to do LLT in a doctor's office.

There are now handheld home use lasers that might work for you if this is a therapy you'd like to try but don't feel like making a heavy time commitment.

Don't count on saving much cash, though; home use handheld LLLTs cost around $300–$500, not a small chunk of change but less than the several thousand you'd spend for in office treatment.

The advantages of the hand-held system are:

- ✔ It's much cheaper and more convenient than driving to the doctor's office.
- ✔ The handheld system, which can part your hair to reach your scalp, may allow the laser to better reach your scalp if you still have quite a bit of hair.

The major disadvantages of the handheld device are

- ✔ You may get tired of doing treatments several times a week, or forget to do it.
- ✔ You may have a hard time judging whether the treatments are working or when to stop them.

Some handheld products emit low level laser when held over your head; theoretically using a comb may deliver the therapy more directly to the scalp. Another handheld system delivers the laser light through multiple clear plastic tips on the end of the instrument that are in direct contact with the scalp.

With this system, 15 separate points of laser light irradiate the scalp. In addition, the floating laser heads of this instrument ensure that the laser light channels conform to the shape of the scalp and head. This direct contact is the main differentiating feature between this machine and the laser comb.

Two of the more popular handheld laser combs are the HairMax LaserComb, which was FDA-cleared (see chapter 18 for information on the difference between FDA clearance and FDA approval) to promote hair growth in men with certain types of male pattern balding, and the X-5 hair laser, which conforms to the scalp arch and delivers energy directly at the scalp level after the hair is separated by the prongs.

Although the manufacturers recommend use of the handheld home devices three times a week, it's not clear what frequency of use is effective, since no evidence has been presented to show the value of either the frequency or the duration of the laser application.

Most of the home use lasers emit a beep to let you know when it's time to move the device to another part of your hair, so you don't laser one area for too long.

In the one reported study of the handheld LaserComb, 93 percent of the participants (ages 30 to 60) had an increase in the number of *terminal* (thick) hairs. In the treatment group, the average number of terminal hairs per square centimeter increased by 19 hairs per square centimeter over a six-month period.

For the same period, the number of hairs in the control (placebo) group decreased by an average of 10.6 hairs per square centimeter, so the relative increase with the laser comb was actually 29.4 hairs per square centimeter.

The base hair counts in both groups were 125 hairs per square centimeter. (As a reference, the average non-balding person has approximately 220 hairs per square centimeter.) During the study, patients reported no serious adverse reactions.

Understanding the Potential Risks of LLLT

We consider handheld lasers to be safe devices that can be used for hair application. There appear to be no safety issues concerning their use and, although the current scientific studies are lacking, they may be beneficial for some people.

One caveat, however, may be that the long term use of LLLT devices for hair loss hasn't been adequately studied, and that long term side effects could show up in the future.

Because some LLLT devices for hair loss have been cleared by the FDA, many people feel that they must be safe and effective. However, FDA clearance and FDA approval are different things (see chapter 18 for more discussion on the FDA's involvement with hair care products).

Obtaining FDA approval is a far more stringent process, with clinical trials required to prove that the drug or device is both safe and effective.

Backing up medical claims

Devices intended for cosmetic use don't generally require FDA clearance or approval. However, one device, called the LaserComb did require FDA clearance because it made a medical claim, that it would promote hair growth in males with certain types of balding.

To obtain FDA clearance, the company had to submit both safety and effectiveness data. The effectiveness data was obtained from a multicenter, randomized, placebo-controlled trial conducted at four sites in the U.S. FDA approval requires a much more rigorous process.

In this study, participants used the laser comb or a "sham" (placebo type) device three times a week for six months. In fact, a major limitation of this study is that the treatment period was only six months with relatively infrequent use, so that the long-term results and safety issues are unknown.

Another problem was that the studies don't appear to have been double blinded (in a double blinded study, the doctors and patients involved don't know who's getting the sham treatment and who's getting the laser treatment) and it's not clear whether the participants may have agreed not to use other treatment modalities, so there's the additional problem of potential biases in the measurement of mean terminal hair density; in other words, the doctor's doing the assessing may have found more hair in the patients who got the actual treatment because they expected to.

Part V
Advanced Hair Loss Solutions

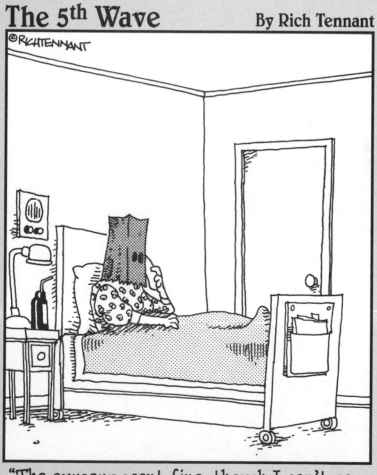

"The surgery went fine, though I can't say much for their post-operative sensitivity."

In this part . . .

When hair loss becomes noticeable, you may feel that it's time to move on to a serious hair loss solution (beyond prescriptions or potions). This section examines ways to hide your head, such as hairpieces, as well as permanent solutions, such as hair transplants. We also tell you the pluses and minuses of both the temporary and the permanent, including everything you ever wanted to know about buying a wig or having a hair transplant — and living with it afterward.

Chapter 12

Hair Restoration Options: Past and Present

Serious attempts at replacing lost hair go back more than 50 years, but great strides have been made in achieving a natural look in just the past few years. Gone are the "plugs" of a decade or two ago; new techniques result in more natural looking hairlines that can make the replacement undetectable.

In this chapter, we look at the evolution of the hair transplant process and explain how the technology, techniques, and skill of today's surgeons can truly restore your hair. You find out about the options for harvesting hair for transplantation, and we also look to the future and the possibility of hair cloning.

Taking the Long Road to Modern Hair Transplantation

Searching for a cure for hair loss is nothing new, but it's only in recent years that greater knowledge of genetics and the chemistry of the sex hormones has helped doctors begin to really understand the causes. *Androgenic alopecia,* also known as *male pattern baldness,* affects more than half the male population to some degree, and it remains the most common cause of balding. Because it also responds well to hair transplantation, hair restoration surgery has gained popularity as a permanent means of addressing genetic hair loss.

Looking at early attempts for a cure

The first documented hair transplant was done in 1822 by J. Dieffenbach in Wurzburg, Germany. He investigated the concept of *auto transplantation* (transplanting from one part of the body to another) using hair, feathers, and skin in animals.

Although there were sporadic reports of hair transplantation in European and Japanese literature during the mid to late 19th century, the modern era of hair transplantation really began in 1939 with the Japanese dermatologist, Dr. Okuda, who used small grafts to correct various hair loss conditions of the scalp, eyebrows, and mustache.

Dr. Okuda transplanted round grafts of skin containing multiple hair follicles from permanent hair-bearing areas into smaller, scarred recipient sites. He noticed better cosmetic results with slightly smaller punches than larger ones in the recipient area.

Here's a brief timeline of key steps toward modern hair loss treatments:

- ✔ In 1943, Dr. Tamura treated 137 patients with non-androgenic alopecia of various causes to restore female pubic hair. He noted that single hair grafts produced results almost indistinguishable from the natural growing hairs. He also noted that larger grafts produced a very unnatural appearance. Due to World War II, the Japanese doctor's findings remained unknown to the Western world.

- ✔ In 1952, Dr. Orentreich performed the first hair transplant for male pattern baldness. Seven years later, he coined the term "donor dominance," which is the basic principle of hair transplantation that hair grafts from the back and side of the head (donor sites) continue to grow hair when they're transplanted to a bald (recipient) site.

- ✔ In 1975, a dermatologist and hair transplant surgeon, Dr. O'Tar Norwood, building upon earlier work, developed a classification of male pattern hair loss that's still widely used today. (You can find more about the Norwood classification system in Chapter 4.)

Tracing the evolution of hair restoration techniques

Hair transplantation began in the United States in the late 1950s. When doctors examined bald men, they could see that there was hair on their heads but it was just located in the wrong places. So doctors became very creative in finding ways to redistribute the hair. In this new field, they used tools adapted from other procedures that dermatologists and surgeons commonly performed at the time.

This section explains the three procedures targeted the removal of part of the bald portion of the scalp and rearranging the existing hair.

Punching out plugs

One of the most popular instruments used in early hair transplants was a circular biopsy punch measuring between 3-4 mm. Readily available, it became the standard way to remove donor tissue from the back of the scalp for the transplant. This hair-bearing tissue was referred to as a *plug* and soon gained both positive (physiologic) and negative (aesthetic) connotations.

Because these plugs were large, skin had to be removed from the front of the scalp (the recipient area) to make room for them. In fact, the same size punch used to remove tissue from the back of the scalp was also used to remove bald skin from the front. It was replaced with hair-bearing circles of skin from the back and sides of the head where the hair was permanent.

This *punch graft technique* was the standard procedure for all hair transplants for many years. It was responsible for the extremely noticeable "pluggy doll" look that people commonly associate with the older hair transplant procedures.

Flapping it over

Rather than punching out pieces of scalp and moving them around, an Argentine plastic surgeon, Dr. Jose Juri, had the idea of directly rearranging the scalp by moving one part of it to another.

He would partly incise a banana-size piece of hair-bearing scalp, keeping one part of it connected to its blood supply. Within a few weeks, the healed flap of skin could be lifted up and moved, provided that the blood supply was maintained on one edge.

The flap was rotated so that the hair-bearing skin covered an area of bald scalp that was removed to make room for the flap (see Figure 12-1).

The defect in the scalp at the donor area was repaired by stretching the hairy sides of the scalp almost to the ears and pulling the two sides together to close the defect, and if the defect could not be closed, the wound would be left open to close on its own.

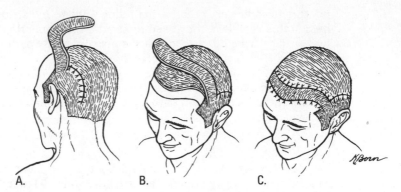

Figure 12-1: A hair flap procedure moved a piece of scalp from one place to another.

A.　　　　B.　　　　C.

This procedure had the following advantages:

- ✔ The results were instantaneous. Other than the time between the first surgery to create the flap and the second one to relocate it, there was no waiting around for hair growth.

- ✔ A hairline with thick hair was created when the flap was secured in its new location.

These advantages may make the procedure sound appealing, if perhaps a bit macabre (moving pieces of scalp around your head?). Unsurprisingly, there were many problems with flaps, including the following:

- ✔ Unless the surgeon was very experienced, the blood supply to the flap could fail, leaving the patient with part or all of the flap dying in its new location in the recipient area.

- ✔ The wounds at the recipient site were often a problem, creating a bald area where there was formerly hair. The new bald area often scarred heavily, sometimes with the appearance of an elevated keloid-type scar or just a scar along the edge of the flap.

- ✔ The hair didn't grow forward, as natural hair in the bald area would have grown. It often grew to the side, or even backward because it maintained its original hair direction in the flap.

- ✔ There was a distinct change from the hairless forehead to a heavy line of thick hair and then, if the patient had any degree of baldness behind the flap the 'island' of flap would be easily seen.

✔ Unlike a natural hairline, which has a slow transition from the bald forehead to the thicker hair area behind it, the flap had a detectably abrupt hairline and then an abnormal transition to baldness on the back side of the scalp.

✔ One flap couldn't cover the entire reconstructed frontal hairline, so two flaps were often used and joined in the middle or off to one side. This produced two open wounds in the area it was taken from (one on each side), two directions for frontal hair growth, and a small (or large) cleft between the flaps.

✔ Multiple flaps often weren't equally positioned, so it wasn't unusual for the hairline to be off balance, with a shape determined by the surgeon's need to cover the scalp rather than aesthetics. As a result, the new hairline of many of these patients just didn't look right.

✔ The flaps were relatively permanent after they were created. The patient had to live with the results, like it or not.

Moving to the scalp reduction technique

The first of the creative solutions to the problems with the flap technique (see the previous section) came in the late 1970s with the scalp reduction procedure for the treatment of balding in the crown area. The procedure was defined by Dr. Blanchard and Dr. Bosley commercialized this technique and published the first large series of scalp reductions. With a business focus, Dr. Bosley created his own terminology for the procedure, calling it *male pattern reduction*.

The essence of this surgery was removal of the bald spot in the top and back of the head. After the bald spot was removed, the surgeon lifted the entire scalp off the head to gain looseness and then attempted to pull the scalp together from the sides to close the defect. Sometimes the defect was too wide to close, so the patient would have only part of his balding spot removed and would return for more surgery some months later. See Figure 12-2.

With a bald area 6 inches wide, it may have taken six or more surgeries to cut out the entire bald area, and the patient was left with an ugly scar where the scalp was put back together. Sometimes more surgeries were required to address stretched scars, and as more and more scalp was removed in successive surgical procedures, the hair on the sides of the head became stretched, reducing the density of the side hair.

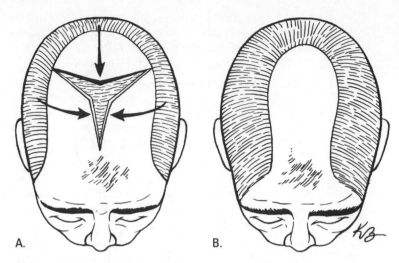

Figure 12-2: Scalp reduction surgery.

The procedure didn't even solve the problem of a bald crown, instead placing a scar in a bald of otherwise normal scalp. This led patients to need hair transplants just to cover the scar and make the crown appear normal.

The scalp reduction surgery was a radical, yet a simple procedure, and the number of surgeries performed spread like wildfire. It could be done in under 30 minutes and cost only $1,500 to $3,000. So the scalp reduction flourished among some cosmetic surgeons, who seemed to forget that patients were paying for the removal of their bald spots with pain, suffering, deformities (see Figure 12-3), and seemingly never ending surgeries.

Although thought to be an attractive solution for the bald male at the time, scalp reduction surgery has since fallen out of favor due to high complication rates, high failure rate with bald spot recurrence, poor aesthetic results, and a disgruntled patient population. This procedure brought out the worst of the doctor's greed for the high surgical fees.

Dr. Mario Marzola tried to improve upon the scalp reduction by dissecting the scalp down to the level of the ears so that more of the lifted scalp could cover a wider defect. With his ability to stretch the sides of the scalp, he was able to remove a wider area of bald skin so the patient would, in theory, require less surgeries. In 1983, he performed the first scalp lift, but to maximize the amount of bald area he removed, he had to cut the nerves on the sides of the head leaving the entire scalp without feeling. Definitely not an acceptable side effect.

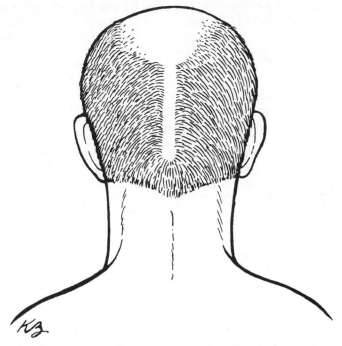

Figure 12-3: Slot deformity as a result of scalp reduction surgery.

Finding ways to produce more natural results

In spite of many missteps, the drive to develop better surgical techniques to move hair around the head led to procedures that were more cosmetically beneficial for the patient.

The usefulness of very small grafts (called *micrografts*) in hair transplantation was first recognized in the early 1980s. These grafts of a few hairs each were mostly limited to placement in the very front of the hairline because of considerable difficulties in handling and placing them into the bald scalp.

A hair transplant that relied entirely on the use of micrografts was first introduced in 1982 in Brazil by Dr. Carlos Uebel. He reduced the size of the grafts (sometimes called *plugs*), but he wasn't able to master the graft survival issues. Although he succeeded in making the results look more normal and natural, the survival of the hairs wasn't great, and the final result looked very thin.

Over the following two decades, transplant surgeons working on ever smaller grafts figured out ways to handle these fragile grafts without killing them. The secret lay in preventing the grafts from drying and in delicate handling during the harvesting and placement process. In refining the technique, doctors came to understand that moving more hair in the transplant would eventually lead to fuller and better aesthetic results. The technique defined by Dr. Uebel evolved into what's now called the *megasession,* large session transplant surgeries.

In 1994, Dr. William Rassman (one of the illustrious authors of this very book) refined the process and published the first medical articles on the megasession. He also started to show off the procedure's results at medical meetings by bringing patients as part of his academic presentations.

In 1995, he demonstrated that grafting large sessions of small grafts wasn't just theoretical, but practical by bringing 23 patients to the International Society of Hair Restorations Surgeons meeting; the patients had experienced considerable balding and had undergone transplants with thousands of very small grafts.

In articles published in 1995 and 1997, Drs. Bernstein and Rassman defined what's now the gold standard in today's hair transplant field: They developed a hair transplant procedure that could, in many respects, replicate nature by moving hair follicles in their normal anatomical groups of one, two, three, and four hairs — the follicular unit in one or two surgical sessions.

Finally transplanting hair as it grows in nature made the results identical to nature's own. This technique they defined is now known as *follicular unit transplantation* (FUT).

The Newest Transplanting Techniques

In hair transplantation, size does matter! In this case, it's the size of the grafts that make the difference, and smaller is better. To make up for the small grafts with less hair, large sessions of grafts became necessary. In this section, we look at the refinements that have made hair transplants less detectable than ever before.

Avoiding the "hair transplant" look

A bad hair transplant is easy to spot. The uneven, patchy effect of large, pluggy grafts occurs when a surgeon uses larger grafts containing many follicular units and the spaces between the grafts are wide. As the grafts heal, they contract and create a contrast between the bald skin and the islands or clumps of hair. Ultimately, the patient is left with a scalp resembling a doll's head.

Larger graft hair transplants took more skin from the scalp, and it produced subtle deformities in the scalp. Skin abnormalities with larger grafts occur for three reasons:

- ✔ The surface of the transplanted skin may not be aligned with the surface of the surrounding scalp. This problem develops in larger hair grafts when the transplanted skin has enough mass to produce the problem.

- ✔ Scar contraction and/or skin dimpling may occur at the recipient site during the healing process. As the grafts increase in size, these abnormalities occur with increasing visibility.

- ✔ As the skin of the graft heals, the melanocytes (the part of the skin that produces pigment) may not recover from the transplant process and give the graft a whitish appearance. This is particularly a problem for anyone with a dark skin color.

Hair in its natural state is composed of hair groupings of follicular units that have one to four hairs close together. In nature, the leading edge of one's hairline is comprised solely of single-hair follicular units with less density than the hair further back on the head. To appear natural, a hair transplant should simulate that look as closely as possible.

To understand the terminology of hair grafts used by different surgeons, hair grafts can be divided into four general categories:

- ✔ **A traditional standard graft,** or plug, is 3 to 4 mm in diameter and has 12 to 30 hairs.

- ✔ **A minigraft** is 1.2 to 2.5 mm in diameter and has 4 to 12 hairs.

- ✔ **A micrograft** is 1.0 to 1.5 mm or less in diameter and has one to three hairs.

- ✔ **A follicular unit** is a naturally growing group of one to four hair follicles. Follicular units are smaller in size than minigrafts or micrografts containing the same amount of hair because the hair exit the skin from roughly the same pore on the scalp.

You should discuss the size of the grafts and the planned distribution of the grafts in detail with your surgeon. Some surgeons use larger grafts for some of their work and then use smaller grafts in an attempt to hide the larger grafts. Others only transplant small grafts.

Some hair transplant surgeons invent unusual terms for grafts to make it appear that they have some special, unique knowledge or technique. These terms are intended to imply special variations in graft sizes or an invisible appearance of the grafts. Don't be fooled by this terminology.

You should be wary when a doctor claims to have a unique technology or technique that no other doctor knows about or uses, unless it's documented and published in a peer-reviewed medical journal.

Small versus large hair grafts

To meet the demand for natural-looking hairlines, doctors began decreasing the size of hair grafts in the 1980s, because of the following large graft disadvantages:

- Large hair grafts are more visible during the transition period after transplantation before the hair grows in. Skin deformities show up almost immediately after the hair transplant.

- Large hair grafts placed in a frontal hairline look pluggy and unnatural when the hair is combed back or to the side. Patients were forced to comb their hair forward and down to hide their hairlines.

- When large hair grafts are placed behind the hairline or in the crown, they look like patchy clumps of hair (even in the most gifted surgical hands) and these are very difficult to disguise or camouflage.

- As healing occurs in three to four mm hair grafts, the grafts contract, pushing the hairs in the graft together and increasing the density of the hair within the graft. The hair density within these larger grafts often exceeds the hair density in the donor area, contributing to the pluggy, stalk-like appearance of traditional grafts.

- Larger hair graft repairs force the patient to undergo multiple transplant sessions in the quest for natural-looking results, and the patient's appearance can be strikingly unnatural until the work is completed.

It takes four to six days for the buds of new capillary blood vessels to grow into the hair grafts from the surrounding tissue. Until these new blood vessels grow into the graft, the graft's cells depend upon the surrounding tissue to bring the needed oxygen and nutrients for their survival.

Hair follicle cells have a very high metabolic rate, and they require more oxygen and nutrients than other cells. If the graft is too large, the cells of the follicles in the center of the graft may die before sufficient oxygen and nutrients can reach the center of the graft. The follicles at the periphery of the graft survive because they're close to the body's nourishing oxygen and fluids.

When hair finally grows from larger grafts, those in the center die and this creates a doughnut configuration, with hair at the edges and a bald central area of skin. This is one of the numerous reasons why many doctors have changed to the use of exclusively smaller grafts.

Small hair grafts also have some disadvantages.

- ✔ The amount of time and work needed to place tiny grafts is greater than what's needed with larger grafts.

- ✔ Smaller hair grafts produce a thinner hair appearance, so many more graft units are needed to produce a natural look.

Minis, micros, and more

Minigrafts and micrografts consist of multiple (partial or complete) follicular units along with the intervening skin. This technique solves the problem of the hairs in the center of the graft dying off, but the contraction of the graft in the healing process still produces a denser graft than normally found throughout the scalp.

These grafts also can cause loss of pigment cells, which can be a particular problem for people with darker colored skin.

Although minigrafts and micrografts are a significant improvement over larger hair grafts, they're not ideal. The idea behind them is reasonable: to keep the number of hairs in each graft low and spread more hair in these smaller grafts around. But the following problems are common with minigrafts and micrografts:

- ✔ Surgeons may move more hair in minigrafts and micrografts, but these grafts appear clumpy if they're not limited to the natural growing groups of hair. Focusing on the naturally growing groups and keeping them intact prevents transplants from looking clumpy.

- ✔ Minigrafts and micrografts aren't harvested with a high powered microscope, so many follicular units are broken apart and the hairs within them are transected during their preparation, which produces significant hair damage and a reduced hair yield.

✔ When minigrafting and micrografting is done with a multi-bladed knife, the hairs within the knife path break up and the naturally occurring follicular units are unavoidably damaged.

✔ Micrografts tend to have more skin in the graft, which makes them lose their skin pigment. Even micrografts containing as few as two or three hairs may contain the skin between two follicular units, which is unnecessary.

✔ Micrografts look thin when used exclusively over the entire head and may produce inconsistent graft growth. Follicular damage also contributes to this thin appearance.

Many surgeons promote a variant of minigrafts called a *double follicular units* (DFU), in which two follicular units are used, each containing one to three hairs. The main disadvantage of the DFU is that there's intact skin between the follicular units, and particularly in the dark-haired, light-skinned, or coarse-haired person, the skin produces a small, white scar as well as cobblestoning (irregularities) on the scalp surface.

This is a subtle change, but one that's visible on close inspection, particularly in bright sunlight. The loudest complaints about such defects come from patients who can see on themselves the points where the transplanted hair exits the skin.

Hybrid grafting techniques

The use of larger hair grafts for the top and non-central portion of the crown and smaller grafts for the frontal hairline and perimeter of the transplant has a variety of names including *blend grafting* and *variagrafting*. Although this hybrid approach is detectable on close inspection, it may not be noticeable in a social setting unless the hair is wet or the patient is in bright sunlight. The results from larger grafts are best in patients with curly, white, or blonde hair.

If you have curly or wavy hair, the hybrid approach or the use of DFUs (refer to the previous section for an explanation of DFUs) may be a reasonable way to reduce the costs of the hair transplant. If you have straight hair, such an approach can be disastrous, particularly if your hair color stands out against distinctly contrasting skin tones (for example, you have dark hair and fair skin). All larger graft procedures generally cost less if the surgeon charges by the graft, and the procedures can be performed without the intense labor required for larger sessions of small grafts.

Another disadvantage of larger grafts may become more evident when further hair loss occurs, particularly when recession allows the grafts to be viewed from a different angle. Using larger grafts or DFUs is more a short-term economic fix than a long-term solution, and we don't recommend it.

Follicular unit transplantation

Follicular unit transplantation (FUT) was the most significant advance in hair restoration since hair transplants were introduced in the U.S. in 1959.

In follicular unit transplantation, hair is transplanted from the permanent zone (from the back and sides of the scalp) into areas affected by balding, using only the naturally occurring, individual follicular units. Drs. Bernstein and Rassman first described this procedure in the 1995 *Journal of Aesthetic and Restoration Surgery*. Because of its superior aesthetic results, follicular unit transplantation soon became the gold standard for hair transplantation surgery worldwide.

 An essential component of FUT is the use of stereo-microscopic dissection — a technique developed by Dr. Limmer in the late 1980s for dissecting micrografts. Applying this technique to FUT, all the follicular units are removed from the donor tissue under microscopic control to avoid damage.

Complete stereo-microscopic dissection increases the yield of the number of follicular units as well as the total amount of hair (upwards of 25 percent). The hair seems to come out of a single hole and that the hairs are bundled together in their naturally growing groups.

The essence of the follicular unit approach to hair transplantation is that the characteristics of the patient's hair dictate the size of the implant (rather than the doctor or the surgical team). For example, single follicular units are placed in such a way as to create the natural look of gradually increased density as you go further back behind the hairline.

Still, the surgeon determines distribution, hair direction, and the balance between smaller one-hair grafts and larger two-, three-, and four-hair grafts. By preserving both the natural physiologic and aesthetic elements of your own hair, the best cosmetic results can be achieved.

 While the term "follicular unit transplant" may be in vogue with most savvy patients and doctors today, not all doctors and their staff have the knowledge or the technical capacity to perform a large transplant made up exclusively of follicular units.

Very few surgeons and practices have mastered the ability to adequately control quality while performing FUT and follicular unit extraction because the learning curve is very slow and the doctor must commit considerable time and money to this endeavor.

Instead, some medical groups may use different graft sizes and hybrid techniques to speed up the process — at the expense of the final result.

Here are some of the many advantages of FUT over mini-micrografting or DFUs:

✔ FUT, when placed in adequate quantities, produces a fuller look because the grafts can be of the same size (or even smaller) than micrografts yet contain more hair and less skin.

✔ The growth is more consistent with FUT than when the follicular units are split up, and dividing the units increases the risk of follicular injury.

✔ Because follicular unit grafts are less bulky than DFUs, recipient wounds heal more quickly. The sites in the recipient area are smaller, making the results look more natural.

✔ FUT allows the surgeon to distribute grafts to mimic the way hair grows naturally in the patient's own scalp.

✔ Because of the greater precision of the harvesting process, FUT enables the surgeon to restore more hair using a smaller amount of donor tissue than with minigrafting, micrografting, or DFUs.

✔ The skin between the follicular groups is trimmed away when only follicular units are used, and the vital support structures around the unit are preserved. Cobblestoning (irregularities in the surface of the scalp) and *depigmentation* (the appearance of whitish blemishes on the transplanted skin) are avoided because excess skin in the grafts is removed, making the grafts significantly less bulky and the holes that they're placed into much smaller.

✔ Because of the very small recipient sites, larger concentrations of follicular units may be safely placed into the bald area, opening the possibility of creating a higher hair density in a single session. More density in these recipient sites reduces the necessity for multiple procedures. The patient benefits significantly with less time devoted to hair restoration surgery without sacrificing the quality of the grafts on close inspection.

With the goal of harvesting follicular units from the back of the scalp without a linear scar, a number of doctors began working on a direct extraction technique. In 2002, Drs. Rassman and Bernstein described their technique, called *follicular unit extraction* (FUE), which we discuss next. This procedure allows the surgeon to remove individual follicular units directly from the donor scalp with a punch of 1 millimeter or less in size instead of a linear donor incision.

This technique, suitable for a select group of patients, eliminates the need for strip harvesting and is a further refinement in FUT. The technology for performing this technique has, at the time of this writing, made significant strides.

Harvesting Your Hair

There are five common methods of harvesting donor grafts, but only two methods — single strip harvesting and follicular unit extraction (FUE) — are used today.

Single strip harvesting

Single strip harvesting removes the donor tissue as a single strip. The strip of scalp is then divided into smaller sections using a dissecting stereo-microscope; it allows total visual control over the procedure and avoids the unnecessary cutting of hair follicles. (We explain stereo-microscope dissection in the earlier section, "Follicular unit transplantation.") The stereo-microscope keeps potential damage to follicles to an absolute minimum, and doctors can preserve the intact naturally occurring follicular units.

The great advantage of this method is that the tissue is removed from the scalp with minimal blind cutting because of the use of stereo-microscopic dissection.

Advantages of strip harvesting under microscopic control is that there's a very high hair yield with an experienced team, and the scar usually is detectable only if you cut your hair to a military buzz cut. Other than the scar and a slightly painful recovery period of a day or two, the strip harvesting procedure is more cost-effective and more efficient from a time perspective. Most importantly, the yield of hair is consistently superior to harvesting without the benefits of a high powered microscope.

The FUE technique can also produce superior hair yields, especially with new technology just being developed. The problem with FUE is that it is very taxing on the surgeon doing the procedure and requires intense concentration for prolonged periods of time to perform the surgery. The surgeon's fatigue becomes a factor when this technique is extended to more than 1000 grafts.

Robotic hair transplantation, presently on the horizon, will use the FUE harvesting technique as its mainstay for harvesting. Robots will not fatigue as humans do when harvesting follicular units and because of this, robot assisted harvesting promises to produce a technology that will be far superior to hair transplantation done by hand.

Follicular unit extraction

Follicular unit extraction (FUE) allows the surgeon to remove individual follicular units without making a linear donor incision and without removing a strip of donor scalp. This technique has evolved into a minimally invasive technique, just like the evolution of surgeries in the brain, heart, joints, prostate, and intestinal areas where classical incisions have been abandoned for most surgeries.

Individual follicular units are extracted directly from the donor area with a punch of less than 1 mm in size. In contrast to the old punch method in which the punch cut out many follicular units in one swipe in order to remove the grafts, in FUE only a single follicular unit of between one and four hairs is removed directly from the patient's scalp.

- ✔ **In the one-step technique,** the doctor uses a sharp punch to surround the targeted graft and then pushes it into the scalp to a depth of approximately 5 mm. The edge is grasped with forceps, and the entire graft is pulled out from the scalp.

- ✔ **In the two-step process,** the skin is cut to a depth of less than 1 mm and then the doctor uses a dull punch to dissect the graft from the deep structures below the skin. The freed graft is grasped with forceps and pulled from the scalp.

The advantage of the two-step over the one-step technique is that the extraction process minimizes (but doesn't entirely eliminate) injury to the follicles in some patients.

FUE has the following advantages:

- ✔ **There's no linear scar in the donor area.** Of course a scar always results from every skin incision, but since scars are very small and scattered in a larger area, they often aren't detectable even when the hair is relatively short.

- ✔ **There are no sutures or staples to be removed.** The small donor wounds are left to close on their own with no sutures or bandages, and they heal within a few days.

- ✔ **There's minimal discomfort in the donor area after the grafts are removed.**

- ✔ **Exercise and athletic activities can be resumed within a week after the procedure is performed.**

Following are some of the disadvantages of FUE:

✔ **Not everyone is a good candidate for this procedure.** Not all doctors agree, but we always test our patients first by taking several biopsies using different FUE instruments and viewing the grafts under a microscope to see whether we can harvest the follicular units without significantly damaging the hair follicles. If we see a significant amount of damaged follicles, we don't recommend this procedure for a patient.

✔ **It's more expensive than strip harvesting.** FUE is very tedious, and every graft should be individually extracted by the surgeon as opposed to the strip method, in which skin is removed first and grafts are harvested under a microscope, generally by a skilled team of dissectors.

✔ **For the same number of grafts, FUE takes more time, sometimes over twice the time, when compared to a strip procedure.**

✔ **FUE produces small puncture scars.** That means that if you shave your head, you may see small, whitish dots. There's no linear scar and the stretched scars of a more traditional strip harvest is virtually eliminated. It is very difficult to detect the FUE scars.

✔ **A large area of the scalp needs to be shaved or clipped very short when a large session of over 600 grafts is performed.** Many patients object to this requirement because of the radical change in their hair styling. In small FUE procedures (under 600 grafts), the areas shaved are generally small, and your doctor will try to shave the areas so that they can be camouflaged by existing hair as much as possible until the hair regrows.

We advise patients undergoing small FUE to keep their hair long enough to cover small shaved strips of scalp. In larger FUE procedures, the shaved areas may be too large to be camouflaged after the surgery. This contrasts dramatically to a strip that can almost always be covered by existing hair immediately after the strip harvesting procedure.

✔ **FUE can produce damage that ranges from cutting of the hair follicles to destruction of vital elements of the graft in the hands of inexperienced surgeons.** The percentage of such damage should be under 10 percent, but that's still a significant amount considering that in traditional strip harvesting surgery, the follicular units taken from the strip under the microscope are mostly perfect.

The Hype About Hair Cloning

Modern hair transplants can greatly improve your appearance, but they have limitations. You can only transplant as much hair as is available in donor areas, and the older you get, the balder you get, so you need to cover larger bald areas with decreasing amounts of donor hair.

But what if you could clone your hair — have one hair replicated in the lab so that it would produce many hairs? The donor supply would be limitless. As simple as hair looks to the naked eye, it may seem that cloning hair wouldn't be all that difficult. There's a lot more to hair, however, than meets the eye. Hair follicles are complex, containing skin cells, fat, blood vessels, nerves, muscles, and glands.

There's also a lot more to hair cloning; potential methods include genetic engineering of the cells, so you never lose your hair in the first place, as well as developing techniques to multiply your own hair cells; we discuss them all in the next sections.

"Inducing" new hair growth

In the late 1990s, a British scientist named Dr. Jahoda took *dermal sheath cells* (cells from the lowest part of the hair follicle) from his own scalp and transplanted them into his wife's forearm. These cells stimulated new hair growth on his wife's arm, and the cells, when analyzed, contained both of the couple's DNA. The fact that his DNA was in her forearm conclusively showed that, at least in this one surgery, he had conquered part of the cloning process.

The results of this experiment have two interesting applications for future hair cloning:

✔ The dermal sheath cells act as "inducer" cells, inducing new hair growth without having to transplant the whole hair follicle.

✔ The dermal sheath cells seem to be immune privileged organs, which means they can be transplanted from one person to another without being rejected.

Even more importantly from a cloning perspective is that "inducer" dermal sheath cells are fibroblasts, which are among the easiest cells to culture. If these cells can be cultured in the lab, a person's own donor area could potentially serve as an unlimited source of hair for the cloning process. That's what everyone wants to hear, but at the time of writing this book, the cloning process clearly isn't there yet. Look for more advances in this area, though!

Some issues and problems to overcome in the area of hair cloning include:

- ✔ Dermal sheath cells are difficult to isolate.
- ✔ The ability to culture the cells has to be proven.
- ✔ The cells need to grow in the right direction — through the scalp instead of under the skin or downward.
- ✔ It's not certain that the induced follicles will continue to grow hair after the initial hair growth is shed (normal hair grows in cycles of two to six years).
- ✔ The cultured cells may revert to an undifferentiated state and stop growing hair over time.
- ✔ It's unknown whether the inducer cells may also induce tumors or encourage malignant growths.
- ✔ FDA testing and approval will take years.

Using genetic engineering to isolate and correct hair loss genes

Rather than replicating a new organism, genetic engineering alters the DNA of a particular cell so that it can manufacture proteins to correct genetic defects or produce other beneficial changes. Genetic engineering involves three steps:

1. **Isolate the problem gene(s).**
2. **Clone (multiply) the gene(s).**
3. **Insert the gene inside the cell so that it can correct the problem.**

The first gene causing hair loss in humans was discovered by Dr. Christiano at Columbia University. She found that individuals with this gene are born with hair that soon falls out (as infant hair often does) but then never grows back. Unfortunately, this isn't the gene that causes male pattern baldness (which is probably the result of more than one gene), but labs are working to isolate the genes responsible for that widespread condition.

Multiplying hairs

In hair multiplication, hairs are simply plucked from the scalp or beard and implanted into the bald part of the scalp. The idea is that some germinative cells at the base of the hair follicle are pulled out along with the hair, and when the hair is implanted, these cells should be able to regenerate a new follicle at the removal site and produce a grown hair at the implant site.

In other words, one beard hair removed and implanted in the bald scalp would produce a beard hair in the bald scalp and in the removal site.

In theory, microscopic examination of the plucked hair could help the doctor determine which hairs have the most stem cells attached and thus which are most likely to regrow. The procedure is called *hair multiplication* because the plucked follicles regrow a new hair, potentially giving an unlimited supply.

In a modification of this procedure, the bulbs of the hair are separated from the shafts and then cultivated *in vitro* (outside the body). After the cells multiply, they're injected into the pores of local, dormant hair follicles in the balding area.

There are three areas where stem cells can be found in the human hair:

✔ Above the sebaceous gland near the epidermis in the upper 1mm of the hair follicle

✔ At the sebaceous gland 2-3 mm down on the hair follicle

✔ Just below the sebaceous gland (the bulge area about 3-4mm down on the hair follicle)

The problem with obtaining stem cells with either technique (hair multiplication and modification) is that:

✔ The plucked cells are only transient amplifiers (cells that grow quickly but for only a limited amount of time before they die out).

✔ The stem cells around the bulge region of the follicle — the ones most important for hair growth — aren't harvested in any significant numbers and can't be readily stimulated to produce a hair.

Chapter 13

Hair Transplant Surgery

· ·

· ·

Surgery can be a daunting prospect even when it's medically necessary, so it's no surprise that undergoing elective surgery for a cosmetic procedure can be a little frightening. In this chapter, we cover all aspects of hair transplant surgery, starting with helping you to determine whether it's a viable option for you. We walk you through the requirements and costs as well as help you find the right surgeon (not necessarily the one with the biggest ad in the phone book). We prepare you to visit possible surgeons and make sure you go in as an informed patient. You find out what you'll face before, during, and after surgery, and we help you be realistic about the possible post-op complications and results that may send you back for additional transplants.

Are You a Candidate for Hair Transplant Surgery?

Do you really need a hair transplant? At first glance, this may seem like a silly question. But hair transplantation shouldn't be your first thought when you start losing your hair. Most candidates for hair transplantation are men with male pattern balding, which takes years to develop. Young men who have just started losing their hair don't know how far their hair loss may progress or how fast. Finding an extra hair or two in the sink or in your comb doesn't mean you need a hair transplant tomorrow — or ever.

Not everyone who's balding is a good candidate for hair transplantation. The best candidates for transplant are those who have the following:

- ✔ Male pattern baldness

- ✔ Enough donor hair to supply balding areas

- ✔ Very little color contrast between the skin and hair color (such as blond hair on a light skin tone, white hair on fair skin, or brown hair on brown skin) if your donor hair supply is limited or you're very bald

- ✔ High-density concentrations of donor hair supply

- ✔ A loose, flexible scalp

- ✔ Hair shaft diameters with reasonable bulk (coarser hair makes for a better candidate than finer hair)

- ✔ Realistic expectations and a good understanding of the process

In this section, we look more closely at who should consider a transplant, who shouldn't, and why.

Those who don't qualify for a hair transplant

Among the people who probably aren't good candidates for hair transplantations are

- ✔ **Most women.** Unlike men, who generally have a permanent donor supply of good, healthy hair on the sides and back of the head (fringe area), women tend to thin all over the scalp including that fringe area. Using a thin donor supply of hair for transplant greatly increases the likelihood of unsuccessful or poor results.

- ✔ **Men with the condition diffuse unpatterned alopecia (DUPA).** These men have an unhealthy donor supply, making them poor candidates for a hair transplant.

- ✔ **People with diseased donor supply for any reason.** This is more common in women than in men and typical for some forms of genetic androgenetic alopecia in women.

- ✔ **Those with low hair densities.**

- ✔ **Those with a tight or inelastic scalp.** This rule does not apply to the 'follicular unit extraction' method of harvesting where the tightness of the scalp is not a factor for hair transplant candidacy.

✔ Those with a lack of adequate funds to continue surgical hair restoration over time.

Those who may qualify and benefit from a hair transplant

A healthy area of donor hair is essential for a good hair transplant, so if you have that, you're already in a good position for the procedure.

Men over age 30 with established male pattern baldness are often more deliberate than others about the decision to undergo hair transplant surgery. They're more likely to have given the matter considerable thought, thoroughly researching the options and finding a doctor they trust. Sometimes a change in lifestyle precipitates the decision, such as a search for a new job, a divorce, or simply the financial ability to indulge themselves.

 The best transplant patients are educated about their hair loss and set realistic expectations for the success of a transplant. They must learn, in advance, the realities of what a hair transplant can and can not do. You don't have to go bald before you go the hair transplant route, but it's best if you're informed and mature.

 Even if you have male pattern baldness, which could eventually be helped by transplant, hair loss at its earliest stage is best treated with medication. The use of medication may forestall a transplant for years.

Unfortunately, young people in a panic may fall prey to unscrupulous physicians whose practices are built on selling hair transplants to those in an emotionally fragile state. Men under 25 years old should think twice before they undergo a surgical solution and should ask themselves the following questions:

✔ Have I looked into other options?

✔ Does my hair loss really bother me that much?

✔ Have I given medication a try and waited long enough to see the results?

✔ Have I thought through the financial implications of multiple surgeries over my lifetime?

✔ What will happen if I continue to lose hair after the surgery is done?

✔ What balding pattern does the doctor think I'm heading for?

It's the responsibility of the physician to make sure that an emotionally distraught patient is making informed choices and understands the long-term implications of any treatment option — especially surgery. With younger patients, it's often prudent to slow down the decision-making process through multiple consultations, stressing the importance of drug therapy, and when appropriate, getting parents or other significant persons involved. Your doctor should allow you to reflect on the situation and the decisions involved — and should never rush to operate. Our rule of thumb for those considering a hair transplant is to delay the decision until they fully understand what it is all about. We tell everyone: A good decision today will be a good decision tomorrow.

Psychological Considerations for Hair Transplantation

Modern society is preoccupied with hair; it symbolizes youth, health, sexuality, and individual style in today's culture. Throughout history, the presence or absence of hair has affected the way people are viewed. For example, during the Middle Ages, men who experienced poor health also had hair loss; as a result, society established biased opinions equating good health — and desirability — with a full head of hair. Unfortunately for some, that public opinion has proven to be pretty persistent.

Balding can make you feel like you've lost control. Hair is one of the few body parts that you can manipulate: You can grow it long, cut it off, wave it, dye it, or pull it back in a ponytail. But you can't control when and how it grows naturally. Hair also serves as a form of self-expression, and as you start to lose it, you may become depressed and withdrawn. Men who lose their hair feel that they've lost control of the image they present to the world — and to themselves.

Hair loss isn't just a physical change. It also has many less tangible effects, namely on your

- Self esteem
- Stress level
- Sex life
- Career choices

There are plenty of studies of the psychological impact of balding but few studies have examined the psychological improvement after hair transplant surgery. Having seen the drastic changes in patient behavior and the high level of patient satisfaction following hair transplant procedures, we decided to take a look at data supplied by mail-in questionnaires we sent out after transplant surgery.

We selected 200 patients who had hair transplants within the previous one to three years for male pattern balding and sent them open-ended questionnaires that focused on eight major criteria. Included were questions on the general level of happiness, energy level, feeling of youthfulness, anxiety level, self confidence, outlook on one's future, and impact on one's sex life. We received 37 anonymous, voluntary responses (an 18.5 percent return rate), which we share in Appendix C. Patients described significant improvements in all eight criteria regardless of their stage of baldness and their ages.

In another attempt to compare psychological changes that patients experienced after surgery to address different stages of baldness, we divided patients into two groups (turn to Chapter 4 for an explanation of the Norwood classification system):

✔ Those who had Norwood Class IV hair loss patterns or less (not so bald)

✔ Those who had Norwood Class V hair loss patterns and above (very bald)

We observed the most significant difference between the groups in the two categories of sex life and career. Transplant had a greater impact on sex life and career in people who had less hair loss at the time of transplant compared to those who had more advanced stages of hair loss. These changes weren't age-related.

Not surprisingly, patients who suffer the most from hair loss are the most likely to benefit psychologically. In early stages of hair loss, patients may be more aware of their condition and be more affected than men in the later stages of hair loss, especially if a patient's hair loss occurs at an early age, when his social life is likely to be more active and more fragile.

Although each individual's motives may vary, it's understandable for people at any age to want to improve their appearance, and hair has a great impact in this regard. However, a decision to proceed with hair restoration should be made with a clear head, a specific objective, and as much factual information as possible in order to establish realistic expectations.

On the other hand, when hair loss becomes an obsession, it's rare that either medical treatments or surgery satisfy the patient's need for perfection. If the patient's emotional reaction to his hair loss far exceeds the degree of hair loss, or if his expectations of treatment are more than can be achieved with existing technology, psychological counseling may be in order.

Realistic expectations are critical before undergoing a surgical hair restoration procedure. Any transplant done in the face of unrealistic expectations is doomed to failure. Realistic expectations for a hair transplant should be based on proper education, emotional maturity, and the availability of adequate finances to undergo an assessment and a hair restoration surgery.

A final result that's more than meets the eye

A patient of Dr. Rassman's is 55 years old and one of the more powerful men in America. If you were in a room with 100 men, this successful businessman's charisma would make him stand out. Powerful and brilliant men and women always surrounded him, but secretly, he felt insecure, not with his abilities but with his aging appearance, epitomized by his balding.

Although his wife appeared supportive of his transplant decision at the time, a few years after the surgery she came to visit Dr. Rassman and said, "I want to apologize to you." The confused doctor asked, "Why do you want to apologize to me?"

She told him about a rift she and her husband had had about his getting the transplant. "I told him that he looked great and that hair wasn't important. But my husband has his own mind, and after the only fight we had in our 27-year marriage, I agreed to go along with him. But I was secretly furious, and I came here today to apologize if I was rude. You see, after the transplant was done and his hair came back, the man I married also came back. I never realized that he could ever feel insecure about what I thought was this ridiculous, unimportant thing called hair. His insecurity was a secret he even kept from me. But when his hair came back, his personality became more open, and his joy of life was enhanced. I saw changes in his passion for life and for me. The contrast was remarkable. I was selfish to think that I knew how he felt, but I never realized how important hair could be. So, I am apologizing to you because I cannot apologize to him."

Needless to say, Dr. Rassman was touched by her apology.

Having Enough Hair for a Transplant

Needing to cover a large balding area with a small supply of good, healthy donor hair can make the hair transplant option a "no-go." Obviously, the larger your balding areas, the less donor hair you have. But you don't need to restore your hair all the way to its original density to develop the appearance of fullness.

For example, uniformly pulling out every other hair (50 percent) from the head of a person with black, medium-weight hair and white skin won't change the person's appearance much at all. At 75 percent uniform hair loss, this person will start to show significant hair thinning, but it's still disguisable with good styling techniques that layer the hair. In contrast, a blond with 75 percent hair loss may show no thinning because of the uniform color of the hair and the light-colored scalp. At 90 percent loss, the black-haired, white-skinned person will show severe thinning, whereas the blond-haired person with light skin color may lose up to 90 percent of his hair and still look reasonably full-haired. It's not fair, we know!

 There's an art as well as a science to the hair transplant process. A good surgeon can achieve the illusion of fullness even when the need for hair follicles exceeds the supply. For example, it's not unusual for the hair restoration surgeon to restore just one area of the bald scalp in a very bald person; putting hair in the front and leaving the crown thin or bald creates a natural-looking variation of a typical balding man who has only crown balding. Viewed from the front, the hair looks normal, whereas from the back the balding crown is visible.

People are born with varying numbers of hair on their heads, ranging from 60,000 to 150,000 hairs. If a man is born with 60,000 hairs and loses 70 percent of them, he would only have 15,000 hairs left, most of which would be needed to cover the areas around the side and back of the head where all of the good donor hair is found.

At the other extreme, a man born with 150,000 hairs who loses 75 percent would have 37,500 hairs on the side and back of his head. Redistributing 20,000 hairs may be enough to cover the entire balding head of a very bald man and make him appear as if he has a full head of hair.

Frontal hairline recession, the most common hair loss pattern, may result in a loss of between 2,000 and 18,000 hairs. Restoring enough hair to replace what's been lost is relatively easy in these cases

Surgeons see less successful results from the standpoint of meeting the patient's expectations when they have considerably fewer grafts to work with. Although the artistic distribution of 8,000 hairs (4,000 grafts) may produce the illusion of fullness, it's a far greater (if not impossible) challenge to create enough fullness to meet any reasonable expectations of the patient if only 2,000 hairs (1,000 grafts) are available.

Planning for Possible Future Hair Loss

Unfortunately, hair loss doesn't stop just because you've had a transplant, so any reconstruction work must take into account what may happen down the road. Your surgeon should develop a master plan to cover any future hair loss; the plan may include drugs like Propecia that slow or stop hair loss. Any master plan should address the following questions:

✔ **What's the worst-case scenario for hair loss in your lifetime?** The master plan should include short-term and long-term solutions. Hopefully, the worst-case plan will never be realized, but it's critical to include this possibility in your understanding of your procedure.

✔ **Will there be enough donor hair to replace future hair loss?** If the surgeon doesn't leave enough hair for the worst-case scenario, then sooner or later you'll be up the creek without a paddle — and without hair, either.

✔ **Will you be able to afford all that's necessary in the future?** The doctor's honest description of possible future needs is crucial to your making an informed, smart decision.

✔ **Are you fully informed about every aspect of the reconstruction process?** We often joke with our patients about changing our clinic's name to The No-Surprises Institute for Hair Reconstruction. Men don't like surprises, and few things frighten them more than surprises in cost or in the achieved results. You shouldn't be caught unawares in any aspect of your hair transplant or future treatments.

Assessing the Costs

Hair transplant surgery is generally not covered by insurance because it's considered a cosmetic procedure, and that means that the cost will come right out of your own pocket. And the price can be high, depending on how much area you want to cover and how much your surgeon charges.

Hair transplant surgeries are generally charged per graft, with a *graft* being one to four hair follicular units. The cost varies between $3 and $20 per graft. Most people focus on the per graft price, as this is how most doctors calculate their fee.

For many people, hair transplantation is limited by their financial constraints. That being said, it's important to look at the long-run versus the short-run when selecting your surgical team. In the short-run, you may save a few hundred, even a few thousand, dollars by going with the least expensive doctor, but if the surgery is performed incorrectly, if the team isn't experienced and loses grafts, or if the surgeon doesn't have the experience or the artistry to place grafts properly, you may end up needing more surgery in the future and worse, you may have a botched job that can not be fixed. The buyer must realize from the beginning that a hair transplant is permanent and errors of design and good planning may not be correctable.

When discussing price, you need to compare apples to apples. One graft (or *follicular unit*) contains one, two, three, or sometimes four hairs. In general, one graft averages about two hairs. Some doctors add to the confusion by charging per hair to make the procedure appear less expensive (this is known as *graft splitting*). Just remember that 2,000 hairs is around the same as a 1,000-graft surgery.

Sometimes a doctor may make single hair grafts by splitting a two-hair graft so that he or she can transplant it to the frontal hairline. But splitting a four-hair graft into two two-hair grafts, or a two-hair graft into two one-hair grafts, just to push up the total number of grafts to make the fee appear like a bargain is the same as double-charging you. Sadly, this is quite a common practice.

Your doctor should be able to explain the exact number of cut grafts and how the numbers were calculated. Ask your doctor how the grafts are counted and to see the sheet that lists the numbers of grafts cut by each technician, because the accounting process of dissecting grafts is highly variable.

If graft splitting weren't complicated enough, you also need to be aware of the "low-ball" sales technique when estimating the number of grafts needed. In this technique, the estimate of the work needed increases after the work has already begun. If your doctor's initial estimate of how many grafts you need sounds low because you sense that he/she wants to make the sale, then you might assume the worst and do some good comparative shopping.

Although the overall cost of a hair transplant is an important factor in making your decision of whether to move forward with it, you also need to have an honest, competent doctor whom you can trust to act in your best interest. The good and bad news about hair transplantation is that it's permanent. Unfortunately, the work of a poor surgeon will be with you for your entire life, so choosing the right doctor and practice is critical.

Choosing a Doctor

The most important factor in hair transplant surgery is choosing the right surgeon. You can have a wonderful plan for surgery, a great medical facility, and marvelous nurses, but if the surgeon doesn't plan your reconstruction properly and then do a good job, the whole thing is for naught. Good planning in how the hair is to be transplanted is as important as doing the technical components correctly.

Basically, what you're looking for is a well-credentialed, caring, competent, artistic (cosmetic surgery is about 50 percent art) doctor whom you like and feel comfortable with. This section guides you through the task of finding a hair transplant surgeon who's right for you and helps you prepare yourself for your office visits to make sure that you get all the information you need to make an informed selection.

Finding a doctor

The best place to start your search for a hair transplant doctor is with friends who have had transplants. Talk with them and look at the quality of their work.

If you don't have a personal connection to someone who has had a transplant, start your search on the Internet. The International Society of Hair Restoration Surgery (www.ishrs.org) lists hundreds of doctors worldwide who work in the field. You also may want to enter "hair transplantation" along with your city and state in your favorite search engine, and explore the results.

Meeting for the first consultation

Going in for a surgical consultation is both exciting and a bit scary — don't lose your head, though, in your excitement about regaining your hair.

Always meet with more than one doctor before making a decision. We also strongly suggest that you look at the Web sites of various doctors, both in and out of your area. The comprehensive nature of these sites will give you a feeling of just how good the doctor is at educating you and sharing his experience and his patient population with you.

This section walks you through what to expect at your first meeting, starting with these first steps:

1. **The initial interviewer, who may or may not be the doctor, should provide you with basic information about the hair transplant procedure.**

2. **You'll fill out a basic medical history form to determine your candidacy for having a surgical procedure.**

3. **Some assessment of your hair loss may be done, but only a physician or a specially qualified nurse practitioner or physician's assistant may legally perform a physical examination and render an opinion.**

4. **A more knowledgeable interviewer may try to determine whether your expectations are realistic.**

In some hair restoration practices, salespeople work at remote offices without a doctor present. These salespeople function independently in many ways and may even wear white coats, implying some medical expertise. If you visit a remote office staffed with salespeople, follow these suggestions:

- ✔ **Ask whether the person you're meeting with is a salesperson or doctor.** Only a doctor can give you a diagnosis and assessment. A salesperson may be able to educate you on the process of hair restoration surgery — and that can be very useful — but he or she shouldn't give a medical opinion.

- ✔ **Make certain that salespeople don't recommend any medical or surgical treatment.** This includes the type of surgical procedures that would be used in your situation, the number of procedures, or the approximate cost of your restoration. Don't accept recommendations without input from a qualified doctor.

✔ **Don't discuss your financial status with a salesperson.** When a physician is available in the office, the patient educator or salesperson should call the doctor in to examine your hair and scalp, quantify the amount of donor hair you have, address your worst-case balding pattern, and then discuss your surgical options. When the doctor reviews costs with you, your cost shouldn't depend upon what you can afford.

✔ **The doctor should outline a master plan specifically for you that addresses future hair loss.** If you can't afford what you need to achieve your goals, ask the doctor whether modifying your goals is reasonable, and make sure you understand the implications of modifying your goals.

It's always best to have the doctor do the entire consultation. During the consultation, a doctor should

✔ Educate you in the procedure.

✔ Take a history.

✔ Do the physical examination.

✔ Discuss your options.

✔ Estimate the number of surgeries it will take to achieve the desired result.

✔ Review all the costs involved.

Busier practices may offload some of these tasks to nurses or clerical people, which may be okay because some of these people will have more time to spend with you answering your questions than a doctor would, but nothing can replace the doctor's advice. One well-known clinic takes the view that the doctor "just screws up the sale" and that it's best to minimize patient-doctor contact. This view is clearly opposite to our thinking.

A good doctor needs to have a strong team behind him. You should expect *physician extenders* to be educated as nurses or certified physician assistants. Doing *refined follicular unit transplantation,* which is today's standard of care, takes a team of 3 to 6 people working together for hours. So, the doctor's team is almost as important as the doctor is. As the old cliché says, a chain is only as strong as its weakest link.

Asking the right questions

Like buying any big-ticket item, buying a hair transplant requires extensive research. A good buyer is an educated buyer, so take the time to do your homework.

First, be sure your doctor practices the standard of care, follicular unit transplantation, in which individual, naturally growing groups of hair are microscopically dissected and moved into the balding area in their anatomical intact units.

When you think you're ready to sign on the dotted line, pause to consider the following questions:

- Did the doctor listen to you, give you enough time to voice concerns, and thoroughly explain the procedure and other options? Did he or she learn about you and your concerns, fears, goals, and economic situation? Did the doctor decide what you will need done to achieve your goals, and are you confident in that decision? Most people can tell almost immediately whether they trust or like the doctor if the doctor spends enough time with them.

- How much experience does the doctor have in the hair restoration field? How is the doctor regarded in the medical community?

- Did you receive documents that fully outline the proposed work? Memories often fail, so the more information that the doctor gives you in writing, the better the communication will be between you and your doctor. For example, did you receive an estimate reflecting the scope of the proposed work and its costs? Many times it takes more than one hair transplant to achieve a patient's need. The patient has every right to know what is in store for him after the surgery. How many more surgeries will be required? The doctor should volunteer this information, but if not, ask about it.

- How does the doctor estimate the cost for a hair restoration procedure? Beware of low-balling — underestimating what you really need to achieve the desired results. Low-balling bids to make the sale isn't an uncommon practice in many industries, but we're talking about what you'll look like for the rest of your life, so low-balling here can have a particularly dramatic effect.

✔ Are you being pressured by hard-sell tactics? Too many doctors oversell, even though it's unethical. Does the doctor keep putting a salesperson between you? Salespeople may sell the doctor's service like a used car. *Note:* Commission sales in this field are illegal in most states.

High-pressure sales tactics tell you a lot about the doctor and his or her integrity. Waiting at least a few days before deciding on a surgical procedure is never a mistake. We tell patients that a good decision today is a good decision tomorrow.

✔ Does the doctor innovate? Is he or she a leader or a follower? All doctors don't have to be innovators, provided that they can deliver a quality service and have learned from the innovators and practice the standard of care. Some doctors misrepresent themselves to build up an image that they haven't earned, such as claiming to be the inventors or pioneers of the surgeries that they offer. With the Internet as a resource, it's relatively easy to verify such claims.

✔ Has the doctor been bombarded with legal problems? Is his or her medical legal record clean? Make sure that you have done your diligence by checking as many sources as you can to determine the history of the medical practice.

Look up the doctor or the medical group of your choice on your state's medical board Web site before making a decision. (You can find a directory of state medical board contact information at www.fsmb.org/directory_smb.html.) State medical boards make available doctors' records with regard to legal matters. You may be surprised at what you learn from the medical board search.

✔ Does the doctor or salesperson try to find out how much money you're planning to spend before giving you an estimate for the proposed work? That's a bad sign. The doctor's first priority should be what is or isn't on top of your head, not what's in your wallet. You should never feel that a doctor is trying to pick your pocket!

Seeing results for yourself

Does your doctor offer patient references? Our office promotes a monthly interaction with our former patients for the purpose of educating prospective patients about the hair transplant process. We also allow prospective patients to speak to someone who's having the transplant procedure and even watch the process.

You can get what you want

A 23-year-old patient had developed the nickname "Captain Forehead" when he first came to see me (Dr. Rassman). His hairline was very high and had receded back about 1 inch beyond his original mature hairline. His temple prominences were set back on his head, and he had the beginning of balding in the crown.

He used a photograph to show me what he wanted to achieve. He earned $9 per hour, had no savings, and had about $3,000 worth of credit card availability. I realized that his goals were well beyond his ability to pay not only for the first procedure he would need but for subsequent surgeries if his hair loss should progress, and I discouraged him from doing the surgery.

Six months later, he made an appointment with my colleague and got on the surgery schedule. I met him again the day after the surgery and was disappointed to find that he had gone forward with a transplant. To my surprise, I found out that this young man had moved out of his apartment and into his 1991 Dodge Omni (he was over 6 feet tall, so it must have been cozy!), where he had lived for the last 6 months. He saved his pennies, got a loan from his parents, and went to Mexico to purchase Propecia long before it was released in the United States. I was so impressed with his focus and dedication that I hired him and put him to work for me educating patients over the phone. This patient now cuts his hair short and no longer looks like Captain Forehead.

There's no better way to evaluate a doctor's work than to see it up close and in person. Good pictures are beneficial, but pictures can be altered or patients can be photographed in ways that really don't reflect the whole truth. When you meet a patient, however, you can look at him or her from every angle! Ask your doctor for direct patient references.

It's best if you can meet with someone who has had a transplant similar to the one you're considering. If your doctor doesn't promote face-to-face meetings, before and after pictures taken from every angle can help you evaluate his or her work.

Before the Surgery

Different doctors have different rules for what you should and shouldn't do before surgery, so always follow your own doctor's recommendations. The following are common recommendations:

- ✔ Ask if you can have anything at all to eat or drink before surgery.

- ✔ If you're on aspirin or any blood thinner, stop taking it ten days prior to the surgery.

- ✔ Speak to your doctor about any medications you normally take, and get instructions about what you should and shouldn't take in the days before surgery and particularly on the morning of surgery.

- ✔ If you're a diabetic on insulin, ask your doctor what to do with regard to your insulin use and your diet.

- ✔ Wear comfortable clothing that's easy to remove.

- ✔ Ask about using an antibacterial soap on your hair and scalp the night before and the day of surgery. If the doctor wants you to use an antibacterial soap, be very careful not to get it in your eyes as it may be very irritating. If you accidentally get it in your eyes, rinse your eyes thoroughly with clear water until the burning subsides. Reducing the bacterial count in the hair follicles is best done with good washing before the surgery.

Review any paperwork you have before you head in for your surgery; this should include all the communications between the doctor's office and you. You should have received a copy of the informed consent form that you have to sign on the morning of the surgery. This document defines what the surgeon intends to do, and most important, it defines the risks of the proposed surgery. You may have questions after reading through it, so jot them down to ask the doctor if anything is unclear.

When you meet with your doctor prior to the surgery, review the informed consent document with him or her. It's not unusual for last-minute questions to come up; legal documents are often filled with every possible risk and can be overwhelming and scary to sign.

Ask your doctor what the plan will be if the actual number of grafts harvested exceeds or falls short of the estimate you're paying for. For strip harvesting, this is a critical question because making the estimation is as much an art as a science. Donor densities vary by the exact anatomic location on the back and sides of your head, so estimates are frequently off by 5 to 10 percent. For FUE harvesting, quantifying the grafts harvested is far more precise because hair groupings are removed one at a time. You can find explanations of these harvesting techniques in Chapter 12.

During the Surgery

Hair transplant surgery is usually performed under local anesthesia, so you'll probably be awake (although somewhat sedated) during your procedure. Often pictures are taken of you prior to the surgery to document your starting point. The surgeon should draw your new hairline on your head; you should have had considerable input into the hairline design and location before this point, because once the hair goes in, it's too late to change it!

The process of determining your new hairline is your last input into what the surgeon will do, so make sure that you've agreed not only on the hairline but also on the distribution of hair.

It is difficult to place a hairline and this process requires a friendly interplay between the surgeon and his patient. There are artistic considerations for the surgeon and there is often anxiety on the patient's part because he must imagine that the hairline that is drawn in crayon, is just a line. The patient usually goes along with the surgeon's suggestions on hairline placement but should voice concerns on location and balance.

After you sign all the legal papers, you'll be given a sedative that should help you manage any anxiety you may have; many patients fall asleep within the first hour of the surgery. The procedure is performed under local anesthetics such as lidocaine or Marcaine injected to numb your scalp and some mild sedation to help the patient through the long surgery. Some doctors use a short-acting narcotic before the local anesthetics are started (like a twilight sedative), and some also add laughing gas to help you through the initial phase of the surgery, when there may be some pain. There should be no pain associated with a hair transplant procedure aside from some small mosquito bite-type shots during the initial administration of local anesthesia. The amount of sedation may be the choice of the doctor or the patient, and the depth of the sedation various with different clinics.

The entire procedure may take place in a surgical chair much like the chair at your dentist's office. Some surgeons allow you to sit up, whereas others lie you flat. You'll be awake, so you can interact with the doctor and staff or just relax — watching a movie, listening to music, or sleeping if you wish. The average surgery takes four to seven hours, depending upon the number of grafts performed and the size of the surgical team.

Most of our patients consider surgery day a great day because they feel good with so many people working on them and taking care of them, and they remain comfortable from the drugs they receive.

Because the day can be long, your procedure may include snacks and meals! In our practices, we serve good food, including shrimp cocktail and ice cream sundaes for dessert, all in the middle of a hair transplant procedure. That's right — you can eat during surgery!

The Night and Morning after Surgery

One of the most common patient concerns after any surgery is what he or she will feel like afterward. What you experience after hair transplant surgery depends somewhat on which procedure you have, strip harvesting or FUE.

✔ **Strip harvesting:** As we explain in Chapter 12, *single strip harvesting* removes the donor tissue as a single strip or oval, and then technicians divide it into smaller sections using a dissecting stereo-microscope to minimize damage to the follicles.

- **Pain:** When you leave the surgical office after a procedure involving strip harvesting, you shouldn't feel any pain for about six hours. Doctors usually administer a long-acting anesthetic when you leave that keeps you pain-free for this period. When the anesthesia wears off, you may have a dull ache in the area where the donor strip was taken. About 95 percent of patients tolerate this discomfort well, but you'll get narcotics in pill form to take home, and we strongly urge you to take one along with a sleep aid when you go to sleep so that you're able to get some rest.

One out of every 200 to 300 patients experience considerable pain on the night of surgery, probably resulting from muscle spasms in the incision area. Your surgeon should give you enough pain medication for this rare occurrence, and you may want to put ice on the bandaged incision area for pain relief. Also, you should be given a travel-type neck pillow for properly positioning the head at home. The pain will usually subside by morning.

- **Bandaging and bleeding:** You'll leave the office with a 1-inch band wrapped around your head, like a tennis sweat band. This puts gentle pressure over the surgical wound, which sometimes bleeds slightly under this bandage. Some bleeding may occur because the long-acting anesthetics contain adrenaline, which constricts blood vessels. Generally, gentle pressure for about ten minutes usually stops any bleeding, but if there's any excessive bleeding, be sure to call your doctor.

- **Next day follow-up:** Doctors generally like to see you the next morning to administer the first hair wash, which is done more aggressively than you may feel comfortable doing yourself. The goal is to clean off all blood and scabs; many patients walk out after the hair wash with minimal redness or indications that a hair transplant was done. The post-surgical hair wash by the surgical staff isn't a necessity, but if you do it yourself, make sure you follow the washing instructions carefully. Your doctor may supply a video to make the process easier for you to understand and follow.

✔ **Follicular unit extraction (FUE):** In the FUE procedure, each follicular unit is removed one at a time. The wounds are less than 1mm each and they are not sutured as they are left open. The wounds swell and often close on their own in a day or two. If they crust, the scabs are very small. Bleeding is usually minimal and healing is very fast, usually in less than a week.

- **Pain:** The best part of an FUE is that there's often no significant pain after the surgery. Patients receive pain medications, but these are rarely needed. The ache that occurs in strip harvesting procedures is rarely present.

- **Bandaging and bleeding:** The wounds from where the grafts were taken are left open and hidden under a baseball hat or bandana. Significant bleeding rarely occurs because the wounds are so small. No bandages are used.

- **Next day follow-up:** Most patients have the option of revisiting the office so that the surgical staff can perform the first post-surgical hair wash, but it's not a necessity following this type of harvesting.

Possible Complications of Hair Transplant Surgery

It's important to remember that a hair transplant is a surgical procedure, and any surgical procedure carries some risks. The risks associated with a hair transplant are minimal, but they're still worth some thought. In this section, we explain the possible complications and estimate their frequency.

We base the following estimations on our own experiences in our hair transplant practices over the years.

Anesthesia reactions

General anesthesia, in which you're "put out," is rarely used for hair transplant surgery. General anesthetics bring risks that are almost non-existent with local anesthetics, such as risk of death or stroke.

Local anesthetics with adrenaline may have effects on many of the body's organ systems, including the heart. Following are some of these risks, along with the percentage of patients that typically experience them:

- Allergic reaction (less than 1 percent of patients)

- Irregular heartbeat (less than 1 percent of patients)

- Heart attack within one month after surgery (less than 0.001 percent of patients)

- Particular sensitivity to epinephrine in patients who use heart or blood pressure medications called *beta-blockers* (less than 1 percent of patients)

- Temporary light-headed episode as a nervous reaction to injections, causing a drop in blood pressure and possible fainting (less than 1 percent of patients)

   This reaction is easily and relatively rapidly treated, most of the time by lying the patient flat and elevating the legs.

Wound healing

Surgical wounds take time to heal. After surgery, any of the following points may apply to your donor and recipient areas:

- Superficial crusting, pinkness, or redness of the recipient area may occur (less than 5 percent of patients), but these effects are usually temporary. In most patients, pinkness disappears in a few days.

- Some area of skin around the suture edges may crust, taking longer to heal (less than 5 percent of patients). A tight suture may cause such crusting.

- A stretched, widened scar is possible, as is a thickened or raised (hypertrophic) scar (less than 1 percent of patients).

Significant scarring is more likely to occur in people who have a history of hypertrophic scars elsewhere on the body (less than 25 percent of patients). True keloid scars (a tumorous type of growth that grows out of the wound and extends beyond the confines of the wound) are very rare in scalp incisions (less than 0.001 percent of patients).

✔ In areas of scar tissue, grafts may grow poorly or not at all.

✔ Temporary swelling, discoloration, or bruising (less than 5 percent of patients)

✔ Formation of a cyst at a graft site (less than 5 percent of patients). Most cysts will disappear on their own, a few may spontaneously pop and drain themselves, and a few may have to be lanced by a doctor or nurse. Cyst formation rarely impacts hair growth. Cysts are formed as remnants of the hair from a hair transplant remain in the surgical recipient site. The existence of such remnants in the recipient sites is very common but cyst formation is vary rare. Usually, any buried remnants are 'attacked' by the body's defenses and dissolved.

✔ Ingrown or buried hairs (less than 5 percent of patients). Ingrown hairs can be difficult to distinguish from buried grafts. A graft that is placed too deeply in the scalp at the recipient site, may sink into the fatty dermis and form a cyst. Sometimes, the surgical staff may place one graft on top of another and this will add to cyst formation as well. Both of these problems may result from staff training inadequacies and problems with in-office quality control processes.

✔ Hematoma (localized blood clot) (less than 1 percent)

Pain

As the anesthesia wears off, if you had a strip harvesting procedure (see Chapter 12 for an explanation), you'll experience a throbbing pain on the back of the scalp, but this can be managed with oral prescription pain medications such as Vicodin or Endocet. Some patients rely on these medications for the first few nights so that they can rest their heads in a comfortable position and sleep. During the day, most patients use over-the-counter pain relievers.

The pain shouldn't disrupt your normal daily functions; most patients are able to return to their normal work activity in two to three days following hair transplant surgery.

Some patients experience pain from the sutures or staples used to close their wounds. Staples are more uncomfortable than sutures but may produce better long-term wound healing. When the staples or sutures are removed (10 to 20 days after surgery, depending on the doctor's preference), most of the related pain goes away. A very small percentage of patients (less than 2 percent) have some discomfort in the wound for weeks or months after the surgery, but this discomfort usually subsides over time.

Numbness

Numbness of the scalp may occur due to necessary cutting of fine nerve fibers in the skin (less than 30 percent of patients). This is expected to gradually disappear over several months, but it's possible that all the sensation may not return (less than 1 percent of patients). This is the consequence of strip harvesting and although it can happen with follicular unit extraction harvesting, it is far more rare.

In extremely rare circumstances, major sensory nerve injury may occur, resulting in long-term or possibly permanent numbness and/or pain in the scalp (less than 0.001 percent of patients).

Having more than one hair transplant procedure puts you at a higher risk of severing a major sensory nerve, which can produce a temporary or permanent sensory defect in the back of the head. Your surgeon's experience is paramount in avoiding this complication. The risk of such damage with strip harvesting although very small, is greater than the same damage from FUE harvesting.

Swelling

A small number of patients experience post-surgical swelling in the forehead if their grafts were placed in the frontal area. In the past, swelling was a real problem for almost every hair transplant procedure, but the use of short-term, higher-dose steroids during and after the surgery has made the problem rarely significant. Applying ice packs or cold compresses to the forehead a few times a day may help reduce swelling.

If swelling occurs, it usually appears on the third or fourth day after surgery and lasts from one to two days at most. You shouldn't feel any pain with the swelling. Most people with swelling look terrible but feel fine. Significant swelling occurs in a substantial number of patients who do not use large dose steroids and less than one out of 40 patients for those using steroids. When swelling does occur, it) usually drops down to the eyelids, possibly closing one eye on the third or fourth day (less than 1% of patients).

Infection

Although infection in hair transplantation is rare (less than 1 percent of patients), you'll be given an antibiotic to reduce the possibility of infection at the beginning of the surgery. Your doctor may want you to use a special antibacterial soap the night before and the morning of surgery to help protect against infection, but washing with a good detergent shampoo may be just as effective.

The symptoms of infection may include:

✔ Swelling

✔ Redness

✔ Tenderness or pus at the surgical site

✔ Fever or chills

If you experience any of these symptoms, contact your doctor immediately.

Redness, swelling, and slight tenderness is to be expected for the first few days after the procedure. If the redness, swelling, or tenderness increases after the second day, you should speak with the doctor. Infection can occur at either the donor or the recipient site. Rarely, one or more grafts may become infected within the first two weeks following the surgery. Infected cysts in the recipient area may appear weeks after the surgery; they look like white pimples or redness around individual hairs. They may be associated with a yellow-colored crust and may be tender. If soaked with a warm compress, they usually drain a yellow fluid following the soaking. If these should occur with any frequency, you should contact the doctor's office. Antibiotic treatment may be necessary if they become infected, spread to other areas, or don't respond to warm compresses.

Almost everyone develops a few pimples in the recipient area at approximately one month following the surgery. These are either new hairs breaking through the skin or the old hair from the grafts being expelled by the body. They occasionally can be confused with a true infection, but pimples tend to resolve on their own in three or four days. As individual pimples resolve, new ones may crop up. You can treat them by applying a warm, moist washcloth at least twice a day for 10 to 15 minutes at a time (you may find it convenient to do this in the shower). If more than just a few pimples develop at one time, or if the skin in a larger area becomes swollen, red, tender, and hot, you must see your doctor to find out if you have an infection and possibly get antibiotics if they're necessary.

Ingrown hairs may cause a cyst to develop in the area of a graft. The cyst can develop over a graft that was placed several months earlier. Cysts appear as local swelling and redness, with or without tenderness. These cysts can be easily treated in the doctor's office.

Preventing Hair Loss Acceleration: Shock Loss

The medical term for the very onerous-sounding *shock loss* is "effluvium," which literally means "shedding." Patients who experience shock loss usually notice it in the first one to four months after hair transplant surgery. Most of the hairs lost from post-surgical shock loss may never grow back, particularly in young balding men.

Hair loss after one to three months may be from a number of causes, including acceleration of the genetic process. Post-surgical hair loss in men is usually seen in the miniaturized hair, and it's possible that some healthy non-miniaturized hair will be shed, but this should regrow. Rarely do patients shed hair from a prior transplant; however, when this occurs, previously transplanted hair that's lost almost always grows back completely.

Rest assured there are things you and your doctor can do to minimize the effects of post-op shedding. Talk with your doctor about your risk for post-op shedding and ways you can reduce your chances of experiencing it, including the following:

- **Use medication:** The drug finasteride 1 mg (which goes by the name Propecia) appears to reverse, slow down, or halt the miniaturization process (when hair is at the end of its lifespan due to genetic balding) and is very effective at decreasing the risk of shedding following a transplant in most men.

- **Time the transplant properly:** If you're experiencing early hair loss but with a significant amount of miniaturization, a minimal hair transplant won't compensate either for potential shedding or for progression of the hair loss. The surgery will have a negative impact in that you may develop hair that appears thinner, or you may have more bald spots than before the procedure, which reflects the miniaturized hairs that have been lost.

> ✔ **Use a sufficient number of grafts to offset any reasonable expected hair loss:** Your doctor can perform a transplant of sufficient size to more than compensate for some shedding.

It's a fallacy that some doctors' techniques are so impeccable that they can avoid effluvium altogether. Of course, bad techniques and rough handling maximize the risk of shedding, hair naturally sheds when the scalp is stressed, and it's stressed during a transplant from the anesthetic mixture and the recipient site creation. Post-op shedding can't be totally prevented.

Having Surgery to Repair Unsatisfactory Results

You have some important considerations to make when considering a repair surgery. Not all hair transplants end up with good results. The major cosmetic problems were caused by the older techniques used prior to the mid-1990s but poor techniques are not uncommon today. Most of the poor results seen today are primarily due to poorly planned or improperly executed hair restoration surgery. Many of these problems are interrelated, and patients needing repair work often have multiple problems to correct. Poor hair transplant work can not always be repaired.

Repairing many disastrous cases is a challenge, and you need to keep in mind that your doctor may not be able to fix everything that's wrong. Partial improvement may still be a worthy endeavor when repairs are needed.

Before repairing a prior transplant, it's important to first establish what aspects of the old transplant work bothers you most. For this, you must clearly express your concerns and priorities.

Some deformities of the transplant that bother your surgeon may be left untreated if they don't necessarily bother you. Setting priorities at the outset will help ensure maximum patient satisfaction. Our most satisfied patients are those who walked around deformed from the old type of transplant work prior to our working with them. Gaining their trust after years of suffering is a major accomplishment by itself.

This section describes some potential problems that may have you heading back to your surgeon for repairs.

Grafts that are too large or look pluggy

Tens of thousands of patients who received the large graft hair transplant technique prior to the early 1990s have the classic doll's head look that people think is what all hair transplants look like. Thankfully, this pluggy look shouldn't occur with today's transplant techniques.

Large plugs placed into a bald head contract in size. Assuming that all the hair survives the transplant, the density of these grafts will (theoretically) be higher than the normal density of the donor hair. So when they're placed into a bald area, they become very detectable because of a pattern of excessive density within the larger grafts and empty spaces between them.

Most patients who have a significant amount of balding don't have enough donor hair to both fill in the spaces between the plugs and cover all the area that needs to have hair. As a result, the surgeon is left with the dilemma of choosing between a pluggy look scattered over a large area or an uneven look, with very high density grafts in some areas and insufficient coverage in others. Often the patient is left with both problems!

When hair is distributed properly in a hair restoration procedure, the density shouldn't exceed 50 percent of your original hair density. The average human scalp has at least a 100 percent visual redundancy, which means that the eye can't perceive hair loss until it exceeds 50 percent of what was originally there. So there's no logical reason to restore more than 50 percent of the original density, especially given that the balding patient has less total hair available. Hair from the old plugs can be removed and redistributed according to this rule or, if available, more hair can be taken from the permanent zone and distributed in and around the big plugs to camouflage them.

The pluggy look may also be tied to less density in the grafts than anticipated from the size of the harvested plug. Two of the most common causes are hair loss from poor harvesting techniques and hair loss caused by a phenomenon called *doughnutting*. In doughnutting, the centers of grafts get insufficient oxygen following transplantation and so the follicles in the central portion of the grafts failed to survive. When part of the hairs around the circle also died, a crescent moon deformity results in hair growing only in part of the periphery of the grafts.

Grafts generally placed without great precision often pit, creating a deep hole in the scalp with hair growing out of it, or are raised above the scalp horizon creating some *cobblestoning* of the skin. Before better techniques were developed and perfected, these unattractive results were common.

Hairline problems

If your hairline isn't placed in the correct position, you won't have a natural look and are likely to seek another transplant to repair your results. Hairline problems fall into one of four categories:

- **Hairline too far forward:** If the hairline is placed too low, it may be impossible to fix. A common mistake of the inexperienced hair restoration surgeon is to restore the hairline to the adolescent rather than the normal adult position.

  Unfortunately, this also occurs when the doctor is anxious to get the patient started with surgery rather than embarking on a more conservative (and more appropriate) non-surgical treatment. A low frontal hairline not only distorts your facial proportions, but also it sets expectations that are unsustainable if the balding progresses. A low hairline also leaves the restoration looking unnatural and unbalanced as you age.

- **Hairline too high:** A high hairline looks abnormal, even if the grafts are follicular unit grafts with single hairs in the front. Locating a restored hairline requires artistry, and placing a frontal hairline too high is the most common mistake of the hair restoration surgeon.

- **Hairline too broad:** Although the adolescent hairline hugs the upper brow crease, the position of the normal adult male hairline is approximately one fingerbreadth higher (1.5 cm above the upper brow crease at the midline).

- **Hair pointing in the wrong direction:** Your own hair direction must be followed exactly for any hope of the transplant looking natural. The only exception is the occasional swirl at the frontal hairline that most likely won't be permanent.

  The hair also must be placed pointing forward, toward the horizon in the front and slowly angled upward as it progresses back. Too many surgeons place the hair in a radial configuration, like the spokes of a bicycle, which is a most unnatural hair direction that never quite looks right. As hair approaches the crown, a swirl is appropriate to allow for changing directions.

  The hair also shouldn't be transplanted perpendicular to the scalp. Although patients are often unaware of the problem, this looks distinctly unnatural. In a properly performed hair transplant, the hair is transplanted pointing forward and then when the hair is groomed to the side or back, the hair is bent, showing the curve of the hair shaft rather than the base.

Unrealistic area of attempted coverage

Hair is a limited resource, so distributing it properly is critical. In the hands of an ethical doctor, there's no such thing as a preventive hair transplant. Areas where your hair still appears normal should not receive grafts. Many doctors transplant behind the targeted bald area in order to push their fees higher, but hair transplants placed in normal hair may do damage to that hair and, in many men, will accelerate the hair loss.

On the other hand, the first areas to bald — the crown and frontal hairline — should be transplanted cautiously, with an adequate amount of hair always reserved for future use. Critical areas such as the forelock and the area behind it will eventually require transplants. If your donor reserves are limited due to poor scalp laxity, low donor density, fine hair shaft diameter, or a host of other reasons, transplanting hair in other less critical areas should be postponed or avoided entirely.

A pattern that resembles two horns and a tail may result when doctors are too aggressive in transplanting the frontal hairline and crown in a young person. This can become a cosmetic nightmare for the patient if he experiences further balding and these regions can't be connected due to inadequate donor reserves.

Ridging

Ridging doesn't occur with the modern follicular unit transplant, but it's a well-known abnormality of the older minigraft and larger graft techniques. *Ridging* is essentially an area of heaped up skin at the point where the plugs were placed into the frontal scalp. This extra tissue makes the transplanted area elevated to the degree that you can see a ridge in the scalp separating the forehead from the area behind. In some patients, ridging is made worse by a reaction of the surrounding tissue in response to the transplanted grafts. This phenomenon called *hyperfibrotic scarring* accentuates the abnormal contour of the transplanted area. Hyperfibrotic changes are rarely seen with very small grafts and haven't been reported with follicular unit transplantation (FUT). (We explain FUT in Chapter 12.)

Scarring

Scarring occurs 100 percent of the time after hair transplant surgery, but if it can't be seen or doesn't impact hair growth, it's not a problem. Scarring can occur in either the donor or the recipient areas. Donor area scarring is pretty much a given in patients whose hair is harvested by the strip harvesting technique, but it may be minimized by certain surgical techniques that can make them almost undetectable in most patients. However, keep in mind that some patients will always scar more than others. Scarring in the recipient area is very rare with modern techniques.

Having a scar removed later may result in another scar in the same place, although specialized surgical techniques may make cosmetic improvements. The degree of scarring after a first surgery where the wound measures more than 3 millimeters occurs in about 5 percent of patients. After a second surgery, this risk doubles. Scars of this size generally can't be seen if the hair length in the back of the head is ⅓ inch or so.

Although the major effect of removing hair from the donor area is decreasing the amount of available hair for use elsewhere, when scarring is severe, the scar itself may become a cosmetic problem. This is most likely to occur when the scar is placed too high (in the non-permanent zone), is placed too low (near the nape of the neck or over the ear), is excessively wide in any location, or is raised and results in a hypertrophic scar or a keloid.

Transplanting hair into areas with severe scarring can cause graft elevation or depression, loss of grafts after the surgery, and poor hair growth. Mild scarring may result in subtle textural and visual irregularities in the skin around the grafts, distort the hair direction, and cause a change in quality of the hair shaft, all reducing the chance of a cosmetically satisfactory result.

Laser hair transplantation, more aptly termed *laser site creation,* represents the epitome of purposeless scarring. The laser is nothing more than a marketing gimmick; it's basically a glorified punch that creates recipient holes or slits in the scalp by removing (vaporizing) tissue. Regardless of how little damage is done to surrounding tissue, the recipient tissue directly under the beam is totally destroyed. (The laser has the additional disadvantages of increased set-up time, greater cost, and potential eye hazards.) Laser operators lack the precise tactile and visual guidance to adjust for depth and angle when making sites on a curved scalp. Most important, the laser destroys tissue, produces third-degree burns, and unnecessarily increases the recipient wound size.

Hair wastage

Careful surgery and a good surgical team using modern microscopically controlled harvesting techniques produce minimal wastage. If your doctors don't use microscopes, the wastage can be 20 to 40 percent of the total hair removed. If your surgeon uses a multi-bladed knife, the hair kill rate may be as high as 50 percent.

Wastage of donor hair from poor techniques leaves you with limited hair for future hair transplant surgeries. Hair wastage may be a result of

- ✔ Poor graft harvesting and dissection
- ✔ Improper graft storage and handling
- ✔ Keeping the grafts out of the body too long
- ✔ Packing the transplanted grafts too closely in the scalp
- ✔ Poor preoperative preparation
- ✔ Inadequate postoperative care

Literally every step of a poorly executed transplant may deplete your donor supply, and all the hair that's lost is lost forever.

An interesting paradox occurs with the old punch-graft technique. When the procedure is done well, most of the donor hair is captured in each punch, but the growth of the grafts appears pluggy, which is a primary complaint from patients. When the procedure is performed poorly, more of the harvested follicles are cut and damaged. Transplanting these grafts decreases the pluggy look and contributes to a softer, more natural look, which initially makes patients happy. However, the poor growth is evidence that there will be problems with hair supply in the future and, ultimately, a worse cosmetic result.

Chapter 14

Caring for Your Hair after Surgery

In This Chapter

▶ Heading home with your new hair

▶ Understanding possible complications

▶ Deciding when (and if) to do it again

Going home after your hair transplant can be nerve-wracking: What if you do something to destroy your expensive new hair? Relax. Caring for transplanted hair isn't that complicated. In this chapter, we tell you what to do and signs to look for in case problems do occur.

Homeward Bound with a New Head of Hair

Postoperative care for hair transplant surgery is minimal; your doctor will explain most of the key points in writing. The most important thing is to keep your hair and scalp clean and free of crusting.

The hair grafts you received should be stable after one day and should be fixed into your scalp, becoming relatively permanent in the few days following the surgery.

 You may notice a small amount of blood from the donor or recipient area after the first day. Just apply direct pressure with clean gauze (which your doctor should provide you with) or a clean towel until it stops. If it doesn't stop with simple pressure, call your doctor.

By the end of the first week you should be back to your old routine, going about your day-to-day activities as if you never had the surgery. If you have enough hair to cover the transplanted area, styling alone may hide the grafts. From this point forward, it's a hair-raising waiting game, as it will take three to six months to see new hairs coming through and about eight to nine months to see 80 to 90 percent of the hair grow to styling length of two to three inches or so.

Recovering after anesthesia

A hair transplant is performed under local anesthesia, just like the dentist uses to fill cavities. Local anesthesia is often supplemented by some form of sedation to keep you relaxed during the surgery. The use of sedatives is a good practice because, like a long airplane ride, sitting in a chair can be difficult for a typical six hour hair transplant surgery.

After your surgery, you won't need to go to a recovery room, but can stand upright and walk out of the office. The effects of the sedatives will last for much of the day after you leave the office, so driving yourself home is out of the question. You need a driver for the rest of the surgery day.

When you're ready to leave the office, a nerve block is put into the scalp; this should keep you comfortable for between four to six hours, after which some feeling and possible discomfort occur. The greatest amount of discomfort occurs the first night after the surgery.

The fear of pain reflects the fear of the unknown. If there's pain, it usually is most intense the first night after the surgery. Your doctor should provide you with medications that help you manage any pain you have.

Keeping your head crust-free

Some patients are afraid to even touch their grafts after a transplant surgery for fear that they may dislodge or damage their investment. But key to good post operative care is keeping the area clean, and that involves some touching.

If your surgeon uses small needle holes for the recipient sites, crusting is minimized and the wounds hold on to the grafts by mechanical means. If crusting or small scabs appear after a few days and persist, this may reflect poor washing techniques, recurring crusting can be minimized by good scalp washing.

Most of the crusting can be removed in the first two days with diligent washing techniques. Here are some of the key points to remember:

- ✔ Never rub the transplanted area.

- ✔ Shampoo once or twice daily. The use of a sponge filled with water mixed with shampoo should be used on the grafted area. The sponge is rolled over the grafts. This rolling motion squeezes the soapy shampoo onto the recipient area. Ask your surgeon for a surgical scrub brush that has no soap in it as this sponge is ideal for washing the grafted areas.

  Never go over the grafts with a back and forth motion as this may pull out the grafts. A back and forth or side to side motion is safe to use on the donor area as there are no grafts there.

- ✔ Washing the donor area can be done more forcefully, removing all blood from the scalp, the first day after surgery. Once all the blood is washed off, the area should stay clean. A back and forth or side to side motion is safe to use on the donor area as there are no grafts there

- ✔ Don't spray water from the shower directly on your head to rinse off the shampoo. Put your hand between the shower and your head and let the water run off your hand until all of the shampoo is off. Pat dry with a clean towel.

- ✔ If the grafts are wet for too long, they may swell and look like they're rising above the skin surface. This will look like little white bumps. This isn't dangerous, but indicates that you're soaking too long. As soon as you dry your scalp, these 'raised bumps' will disappear as the grafts settle down and the swelling goes away.

- ✔ If the crusts appear larger than the grafts because of bleeding that may have occurred the first night, try to get these crusts off by rolling a moist cotton swab over the crust. Don't wipe it, just roll it, as the cotton fragments will gently pull pieces of the crust off. You need to be very gentle, so repeat the process over and over again until the crusts disappear. You don't want to force any of the grafts out.

- ✔ The grafts are usually securely locked in place by the fifth day if the areas has been kept crust free. If the crusts last longer than five days, it means that you haven't washed vigorously enough. Vigorously pulling or scrubbing crusts that remain after five days can cause the crusts to pull the grafts out.

WARNING!

The rule of thumb we use is that grafts must be crust free to be considered secure. Grafts can come out for up to 12 days after surgery if crusts are present and you scrub them or pick at them. This is an important rule because patients are worried that they will pull out the grafts by something that they do.

The photo on the left in Figure 14-1 was taken an hour after a hair transplant surgery of 1500 grafts (note that there's no crusting or bleeding present, because the recipient site holes were very small).

The photo on the right was taken 11 days after the surgery. At no time did the patient have scabs or crusting on the recipient area. This is the typical post-operative appearance of our patient surgeries. This patient went to work on the second post operative day without any detection by his colleagues because he managed the washing properly.

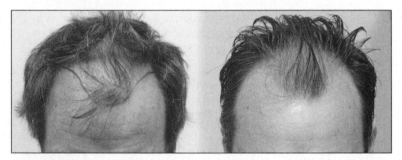

Figure 14-1: Typical postoperative appearance one hour after surgery (left) and 11 days later (right).

Hiding your head

It's always nerve wracking walking into a crowd with a new look, and it's especially nerve wracking when you're worried that everyone is going to be whispering behind your back, "Did he or didn't he?" While it's normal to be self conscious at first, there are ways to detract attention from your head and to hide your surgery from the curious and the nosy!

If you have enough hair to cover the transplanted area, styling alone may hide the transplants. From this point forward, it's a hair raising waiting game, as it will take three to six months before you see new hairs coming through, and about eight to nine months to see 80 to 90 percent of the hair growth to styling length of two to three inches or so.

If you're very bald and concerned that someone may notice your transplant, try growing out your beard! Don't shave starting the day prior to the transplant and let your beard take on a stubbly look. The change to your face will divert eyes from your scalp; even a very bald man can hide the transplant with this technique.

For men with beards or mustaches, try shaving them off. This will always produce comments about your new look and again will divert attention from the top of your head!

Keeping your hair long before surgery is very important because long hair can be styled to hide all of the wounds on the back and side of the head (where the donor was removed).

As the recipient graft site will initially feel like beard stubble and will grow over the next day and thereafter, the short transplanted hairs will hold all of the long hair that is combed over it in place without hair spray.

The beard-like recipient hairs will look like they're-growing out for the first two weeks or so and then they usually fall out. Don't panic at this! It doesn't mean that you've lost these precious hairs, but that the hair has entered its telogen (rest) cycle, which may last up to five months before the hair begins to reappear.

Limiting your amount of exercise

With regard to strip harvesting, you can play golf or tennis by the second day after surgery (your swing may be off because of the pull of the sutures or staples), or you can even run a marathon one week later. The main concern with postoperative exercise is the stress on the donor areas on the scalp from which grafts were taken. For example, straining or stretching the back of the neck (e.g. pull-ups or sit-ups) may lead to a wider scar and should be avoided.

It's good to walk and exercise within a few days after a transplant. Because the impact of exercise varies greatly from person to person, we can't make hard and fast recommendations; be sure to discuss your particular concerns with your doctor.

With regard to FUE harvesting wounds, there are no exercise restrictions after a week. (See Chapter 12 for more on the types of hair plant surgeries.) The same washing techniques discussed above, must be applied to the recipient area and the donor area can be washed vigorously after the third day. The donor area, however, can be scrubbed vigorously after three or four days.

Sutures or staples can be removed between 9 and 17 days after surgery depending upon the surgeon's assessment of your healing. Staples tend to be more uncomfortable than sutures, but they may produce better wound healing than sutures in the long run.

For strip harvesting wounds, exercises that don't flex the neck or put pressure on the back of the neck are usually okay. You may resume swimming three weeks after your procedure, but you shouldn't soak the donor wound for a full month.

In general, exercises such as sit-ups (especially with your hands clasped behind your head), squats, heavy weight-lifting, and bench presses strain the back of the neck and should be avoided for at least four weeks following surgery. If the back of the scalp feels tight after four weeks, or if you have a tendency to heal with wide scars, you should avoid these activities for three to six months.

For FUE harvested areas, you can resume swimming in one week provided that the wounds are all closed by that time; there are no restrictions for any other form of exercise.

The donor wound won't regain its full strength from strip harvesting for at least three to six months after the surgery, so use a reasonable degree of caution during this period. Use good judgment, and call your surgeon if you have questions.

Handling Complications

As with any surgery, hair transplantation can have complications even past the normal postoperative period. This section reviews some of the potential problems to be aware of following your surgery.

Post operative brow and facial swelling

With all head and scalp surgery, swelling is common. At times the swelling can be very significant, causing an eyelid to swell shut. When swelling appears, it usually occurs on the third or fourth day and lasts only one or two days.

Most post operative swelling can be eliminated with the judicious use of large doses of steroids started the day of surgery and taken over four to five days. The use of steroids, however, must be carefully weighed since certain medications or medical conditions may prohibit their use, such as diabetes, which tends to be aggravated with steroid use.

Your surgeon will need to make the call on whether steroids are worth the potential complications in your particular case in collaboration with your medical doctor.

Failure of transplanted hair to grow

As with all surgical procedures, results from hair transplants can't be guaranteed. It's possible that some or all of the transplanted hair may fail to grow (this occurs in less than one percent of cases). Every effort will be made to give you the maximum yield from your transplanted hair.

Alopecia Areata (AA), or spot baldness, can in rare cases exist in a diffuse form that resembles genetic balding. The diffuse form of this disease, when it occurs, is more frequent in women than in men, and can be a cause of a transplant failure if your body's immune system attacks the hair follicles (<0.1 percent chance). AA can be diagnosed by multiple biopsies.

Failure of the transplants to grow can be caused by other factors such as technical failures by the surgical team, due to inexperience and/or sloppy surgical methods. We call this the H (human) factor. As this surgery is a team effort, the team is only as good as its weakest member. Inexperience in the surgical team is the most probable cause of graft growth problems.

On rare occasions, the grafts may not all grow, even though your surgeon and the surgical team do everything perfectly. The hair transplant industry has called this the X factor, which simply means that there's no identifiable cause for the problem.

Clearly X factor is an additional set of factors beyond the patient's scalp condition or the surgical team. The chances of failure to grow from X factors should be less than one percent in the hands of an experienced surgical team.

When hair fails to grow, it may be helpful to biopsy the scalp in the areas where the failure occurred, but because this type of failure is so unusual, biopsies are not recommended in advance of the transplant.

Hair loss

Hair loss can occur at both the recipient site and the donor site. For men, hair loss at the recipient site is related to genetic induced miniaturization of the existing hair and minimized by taking finasteride (1 milligram daily). This drug is effective fairly quickly (in the first 24 hours).

Young men are at greater risk for post operative hair loss so a daily dose of finasteride is important to prevent what is referred to as *shock loss* or accelerated thinning secondary to the genetic balding process. (The next section explains shock loss.) If you're a man under 35, planning hair transplant surgery, you should talk to your doctor and begin taking finasteride at least two weeks prior to the procedure.

Men over age 35 have less chance of shock hair loss after a hair transplant because their genetic hair loss has usually slowed by that age.

When hair loss occurs in the recipient area in a young man with genetic hair loss who has not been on finasteride, the loss may be permanent. This type of loss usually occurs in the first six months post surgery. When hair loss occurs in women in the recipient area, the loss is rarely permanent, but it may take four to six months for hair to regrow in the recipient area.

Hair loss can also occur around the donor area; this is most often the result of a wound closure that's too tight. When hair loss occurs in the donor area, it usually starts at about ten days after surgery and completes its course over the following six weeks.

When hair falls out in the donor area, it usually re-grows over the ensuing four to eight months. The hair that is shocked is forced into its sleep (telogen) phase, but will usually recover.

Hair loss acceleration: Shock loss

While hair loss after transplant is always a shock, shock loss refers to a specific type of post surgical hair loss. Turn to Chapter 13 for more about shock loss, what it is, how often it occurs, and what can be done about it.

Surgery and the anesthesia associated with the surgery can stress hair so that the hair might continue its loss on an accelerated time-line. We see this in men and women (see Chapter 13).

Sun damage

After your transplant, you must protect your scalp from the damaging rays of the sun, particularly for the first three months. Although sun will not prevent the new transplanted hair from growing, it can damage the healing process. Ultraviolet light damages newly formed collagen. If you have a history of skin cancer or sun-damaged skin, you should follow up regularly with your dermatologist.

It's possible that significantly sun-damaged skin may hinder hair growth because the blood vessels of the scalp can be damaged.

Wear a hat to protect yourself in the sun. After the scabs or crusts have fallen away, you can (and should) apply sunscreen to the scalp.

Doing It Again

If you feel that you need more hair, more fullness, you may want to consider another surgical hair transplant. You should wait a minimum of eight months after the previous procedure, when 80 to 90 percent of the transplants will have grown out. You need to see the results of your transplant before making a decision to have another. Ask yourself the following questions as you ponder a second surgery:

- ✔ Have you achieved your goals?
- ✔ Did the hair transplants cover the balding area you wanted to cover?
- ✔ Is the hair full enough?
- ✔ How did the wound heal? Is it detectable?

Many fairly bald patients or those with fine hair should expect to have more than one procedure for the best results. Still, it's possible that you'll feel that you've achieved your goal in one session and don't feel that more hair will add value to your results. See Chapter 13 for more.

Part VI
The Part of Tens

The 5th Wave   By Rich Tennant

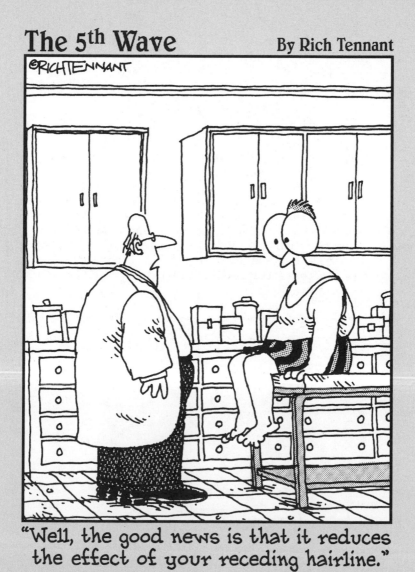

"Well, the good news is that it reduces the effect of your receding hairline."

In this part . . .

*W*ondering which myths about hair loss are true and which ones aren't? Looking to weigh the advantages and disadvantages of hair replacement surgery versus hairpieces? Want to know more about how the Food and Drug Administration (FDA) looks out for your interests — and what it doesn't do — when approving new medications and medical devices related to hair loss? We cover these topics in this section, which is chock-full of easy to access and easy to digest info to answer all your lingering questions.

Chapter 15

Ten (or so) Myths about Hair Loss

In This Chapter

▶ Debunking myths about the causes of hair loss

▶ Revealing what doesn't prevent hair loss

*B*ecause people are so attached to their hair (pun intended), a number of myths have sprung up regarding hair — when and why it goes gray, what causes baldness, and how baldness can be prevented are just a few topics of focus. Wherever people are going bald or worried about losing their hair, myths about hair abound. This chapter turns an objective eye to hair myths so you can separate the serious from the silly when it comes to hair loss.

Hair Loss Comes from Your Mother's Side

The idea that you inherit a baldness gene only from your mother's side of the family is a myth. The inheritance of common baldness appears to be found on the autosomal — the non-sex-related — chromosomes, which means that baldness can come from either parent. Moreover, the baldness gene is a dominant gene, meaning that you need only one gene on one chromosome to express the balding trait, although multiple genes appear to influence the balding process.

You can get some insight into baldness by examining balding patterns in your relatives. If you have an uncle, father, or grandfather who's bald or balding, find out when he started to lose his hair; it may be an indication as to when you may go bald. Just don't put all the blame on Mom if you start to lose your hair. It's not her fault!

Women also inherit the thinning or balding patterns found in their families, but the patterns that are inherited are distinctly women's patterns, not men's pattern. This suggests that the inheritance patterns in women do not follow the inheritance patterns in men. Women with hair loss or thinning will frequently report that they take after their mom, grandmother (either side of the family), sister, aunt, etc.

Wearing Hats Causes Hair Loss

More than a few people believe that hats are to blame for baldness based on the idea that hats cut off air circulation to the scalp and prevent the scalp from breathing. What they don't know is that hair follicles get oxygen from the bloodstream, not the air, so you can't suffocate your hair follicles just by wearing a hat. The baseball cap so often worn by men whose hair is thinning doesn't cause baldness — it hides baldness.

Hats that fit *tightly* on the head are another story. These hats may cause thinning around the sides of the head where constant traction is applied to the hair. Hats worn all the time for cultural and religious reasons (such as turbans and yarmulkes) may cause hair loss, too. In rare cases, sports helmets have been known to cause traction alopecia in athletes who wear their helmets too often, particularly if the helmet rubs repeatedly against an area of the scalp, causing "traction."

If You Don't See Hair in the Drain, You Aren't Balding

You don't go bald because your hair is falling out; you go bald because your normal, thick hair is gradually being replaced by finer, thinner hair in a process called *miniaturization*. Yet people who are sensitive to the prospect of going bald often obsessively scrutinize the shower drain and the hairbrush for evidence of impending baldness.

Most people lose about 100 hairs daily but grow another 100 hairs daily to replace what's lost. Some of the lost hairs wind up in your shower drain or hairbrush, or they may just fall off as you go about your normal activity, responding to whatever your environment dishes out.

Risking it all to cover up

Many of Dr. Rassman's patients have lived underneath baseball caps for years, never venturing outside without them. The best example is Sam, who was in the shower when the 1994 Northridge earthquake hit in California. Sam never went out without his baseball cap, but when his apartment started to shake, he put a towel around his waist and ran out of the apartment without his baseball hat on. When he reached the street half-naked, Sam realized his head was also naked and immediately ran into the shaking building to retrieve it. He returned to the street still wearing only his towel — but he had his baseball cap!

Dr. Rassman's office has many Open House events, and Sam comes to many of them to share this story with the audience of prospective hair transplant candidates and to show off his glorious hair. He never wears a baseball cap since finishing his transplant reconstruction.

Massive hair loss appearing in the shower drain should alarm you (as should a trail that forms behind you as you walk down the hall!), but insidious, progressive loss may be far more subtle. If progressive loss persists over time, you may lose far more hair than you'll ever see in the shower drain. This is particularly the case with female hair loss.

Excessive Use of Hair Chemicals and Hot Irons Kills Your Hair

Hair isn't alive, so hair products or hot irons can't "kill" hair, although they may cause hair damage. As long as the damage caused by hair products is limited to the hair and not the growing hair follicles below the skin, hair above the skin may be lost from breakage or damage, but it will re-grow from the follicles at a rate of ½ inch per month.

Damaging hair follicles below the skin, however, can cause baldness. When inexperienced people apply chemicals such as unsafe dyes or relaxing agents to the hair and scalp, the caustic chemicals may work their way into the growing part of the hair follicle and damage or kill the hair follicle at its root. The longer powerful chemicals stay on the scalp, the deeper they may penetrate into the pores of the skin where the hair follicles are, resulting in permanent hair loss or hair that may never look "healthy."

Applying dyes, chemicals, or hot irons (even hair rollers that are too hot) can cause the hair to become fragile and break off. Hair breakage and split ends are most common in people with long hair because the hair is around for a longer amount of time before being cut, so it's more susceptible to damage from wind, drying, and sunlight as well as chemicals such as relaxers and hair dyes.

Hair Loss Is Caused by Decreased Blood Flow

One hair loss myth says that standing on your head increases the flow of blood to your scalp and thereby improves hair regrowth and regeneration. Although the act may entertain the neighbors and give you a unique look on life (albeit an upside-down one), specialists agree that standing on your head has no impact whatsoever on hair loss. Growing hair does require a significant amount of blood flow, but after you lose hair, blood flow to your scalp decreases because, well, you just don't need it with no hair up there.

There's a cause and effect issue here, but it's important to remember that the hair loss occurs *before* the blood flow decreases. Decreased blood flow to the scalp isn't the cause of the hair loss but rather the result of it. The absolute proof of this is that, when good hair is placed into a bald scalp with decreased blood flow, the blood flow returns when the hair starts growing.

Magnets Increase Hair Growth

In the early days of electricity, magnetic devices were commonly sold in local newspapers as a cure for hair loss. Magnetic therapy, a kind of alternative medicine, holds that magnetic fields can yield health benefits by improving blood flow. Backers of the therapy claim that it can be used to treat arthritic joints, circulation problems, and erectile dysfunction.

Over the years, we've been asked many times whether magnets can increase hair growth. The answer is a definitive "no." Even if magnetic fields do affect blood flow — and that's a dubious proposition — increasing blood flow to the scalp doesn't prevent hair loss or regenerate hair.

Brushing Your Hair Is Better Than Combing It

When you tug and pull a comb or brush through the tangles and knots in your hair, you may pull out a few hairs, but they'll grow back because brushing and combing healthy hair doesn't disturb the hair follicles below the skin surface. Brushing the hair isn't necessarily better than combing because the real issue is *how* you brush or comb the particular kind of hair you have. Tugging on knotted hair isn't good even for healthy hair, but hair that has already started being miniaturized is more susceptible to loss from any kind of rough treatment, including that with a comb or brush.

 You're less likely to damage your hair using a wide-tooth plastic comb or a brush as opposed to a metal comb or one with finer, tighter teeth; these combs tend to be rougher and more traumatic to the hair shaft. When brushing or combing, direct your motion in the direction of hair growth so that the hair shaft (the grain of the hair) is in line with your brushstrokes.

Cutting or Shaving Your Hair Make It Grow Back Thicker

Getting frequent haircuts doesn't make your hair grow more thickly, but it's easy to see how this particular myth came about. When hair is cut short, it gets scratchy like sandpaper, and when you run your fingers through this scratchy hair, it seems thicker than it did before. But it's not thicker — it's just shorter. Hair grows on average at a rate of a ½ inch per month. It grows at that rate whether you cut it daily or get a haircut only during leap years on February 29.

Hair Loss Is Caused by Clogged Pores

Many dishonest people claim that clogged pores are the cause of hair loss. Some folks build huge businesses around massaging hair and "treating" the clogged hair follicles to allow the hair to come through the skin. From my experience, people who sell such services command a healthy price between $200 and 500 per month.

If common baldness were simply due to clogged pores, you wouldn't need anything more than rigorous shampooing to maintain a full head of hair. But I'm sure you've seen men and women who don't wash their hair often but who don't seem to have a problem with balding.

Men in particular buy into this clogged pore myth because they feel helpless at watching their hair fall out; when someone tells them that frequent massage and the use of special lotions will free up these clogged pores, they buy into it hook, line, and sinker. Of course, they do get some reward because the head massage feels great.

Frequent Shampooing Causes Hair to Fall Out

When you notice your hair starting to thin, you may blame your shampoo. You notice shed hair in the bathtub or shower and decide to shampoo less often to keep from losing hair. As a result, hair that would normally come out in the bath or shower builds up on the scalp. With the next shampoo, you see even more hair loss, confirming your original suspicion that shampooing causes baldness. Thus another hair myth gains footing.

Hereditary baldness isn't caused by hair falling out but by normal hair gradually being replaced by finer, thinner hair. Shampoo has nothing to do with baldness.

Hair Loss Stops When You Get Older

This myth is partly true because hair loss slows down in men as they age. Usually, men over the age of 60 see only marginal loss, if they have any hair loss at all. For women, the exact opposite is true: with age and the loss of the protective hormone estrogen, women with genetic hair loss find that the hair loss process that starts during menopause gets progressively worse as they age.

Chapter 16

Ten Pros and Cons of Non-Surgical Hair Replacement

In This Chapter

▶ Appreciating the advantages of hair replacement systems

▶ Weighing the disadvantages of hair systems

*U*sing a so-called "hair system" (discussed in full detail in Chapters 6 and 7) isn't for everyone, but considering that non-surgical hair replacement is a multibillion dollar industry, it's clearly the right decision for many. Despite the common stigma and jokes about "rugs" or "mops," a good hair system isn't easy to detect, can be easy to use, and can help cover extensive hair loss problems and other scalp deformities. A good hair system also can be a good solution for temporary hair loss. As with most things in life, there are pros and cons to hair replacement systems. In this chapter, we weigh them out for you.

The Pros of Hair Replacement Systems

Hair systems have definite advantages to some people in some situations. In this section, we share three of the most common reasons that people get hair replacement systems.

The immediate change

One great thing about a hair replacement system is that the results are instantaneous. Put it on your head, and you can see exactly what you'll look like a week, a year, or ten years from now. You don't have to wait for a wig to grow, or worry that it might not "take" like a hair transplant or a medical therapy. Hair systems are sure things.

You can buy hair replacement systems in multiples, which means you can change your look easily and have a spare if something should happen to one system.

Quick solutions to mask medical problems

With some patients, such as men who have very advanced hair loss where their supply of donor hair is inadequate, or people with various forms of autoimmune diseases (see Chapter 5), surgical restoration or other hair replacement alternatives are impossible. In these cases, hair systems can be an excellent choice.

Men and women who have temporary hair loss resulting from chemotherapy often opt to wear wigs. In diseases such as *alopecia totalis,* which causes total loss of hair on the head, only a full helmet-type wig works. Wigs are also an excellent cosmetic solution if you have extensive patchy *alopecia areata,* an autoimmune condition that results in partial, often temporary hair loss.

Using a hair system as a temporary solution for a temporary problem is invaluable. If you need to wear it for an extended period of time, you can attach a wig with tape or glue in the same manner as a smaller hair system. "Vacuum-fit" attachment devices designed especially for full scalp, helmet-fitting wigs offer the benefit of a very secure but not a very comfortable fit (as these vacuum hair systems are a helmet in size, they are equipped with a suction device to hold the helmet in place.) Keep in mind, though, that many of these helmet type hair systems don't "breathe" and can be hot, particularly in the summer.

Initially lower cost

We can't argue that over a lifetime, replacing, repairing, washing, and otherwise fooling around with wigs can be more expensive than having a hair transplant, but the initial cost is still lower. Many people opt for wigs instead of transplants, accepting the long-term costs, for any or all of the following reasons:

- They can't afford the high initial cost of a hair transplant. For many people, a few thousand dollars a year is easier to swallow than tens of thousands all at once.

- They're scared to death at the thought of having surgery.

> ✔ They anticipate a day when they won't wear a hair system.
> After ten years or so, or when a person ages to a point where
> vanity isn't such a big issue, he or she (more commonly "he")
> may decide it's time to go "au natural."

The Cons of Hair Replacement Systems

Using a hair system isn't without its disadvantages. You may find
that these negatives far outweigh the positives, or you may find
that the opposite is true for you. Regardless, there's no fault in a
well-informed decision, so this section lays the disadvantages of
hair systems on the line.

Living with the fear of discovery

There's great fear among hair system users that the system may be
too obvious and detected. Although there's no such thing as a
completely detection-free and worry-free hair system, high quality
ones can look very real. But they're often very expensive and require
careful and constant upkeep. Because most people feel that a hair
system is a cover-up, you must be ever aware of the status of your
hair system: where it's located on the head, how firmly the attachment is, and how well-groomed it is.

Depending on the size and shape of your hair replacement system,
you may need to have it styled just like your own hair in order to
make sure it blends in and goes undetected. Although the piece
won't grow, the hair around and beneath it will, so you must have
your natural hair cut frequently to match the length of the hair
system. Blending the two maximizes the natural look of your whole
head of hair. The thickness of your hair and the thickness of the hair
of the hair system should also be similar (although they rarely are).

If your hair system covers a substantial portion of your head, you
must decide what to do with the normal hair under the hair system
(if you have some). If you decide to shave it, you can attach the
system with glues or tapes. If you keep your normal hair long, clips
or weaves may be the best way to attach the system.

What makes a hair system detectable? One of the most common
errors in selecting a hair system is ignoring the frontal hair line.
People see the frontal view first, so it's where you're most vulnerable. With natural hair, the frontal hairs create a delicate transition

zone from the bald forehead to the thick hair behind it, usually covering a distance of about ½ inch. The challenge with a hair system is recreating that zone with fine, skin-matched mesh extension with fine hairs in front of the thicker hair of the hair system. The mesh drives up the cost considerably, so many people just accept the hair system without a frontal extension.

One way to blend the frontal view without a fine mesh extension is to buy a hair system that has internal cover for the frontal hairline and use styling tricks, such as a side-combed style shifted forward, to hide the actual hairline.

Chasing the fly-away wig

When you wear a hair system, by far your worst nightmare is that a sudden wind may sneak up behind you and blow the hair right off of your head (we call this the "fly-away wig"). More commonly, the attachment moves because it comes loose as a result of hair growth under the bonding system where the system is physically attached. The bonding can become loose as the outer layer of skin starts to slough, or it may just start to break down.

Frequent upkeep takes the stress out of the problem of "keeping your hair on." Pay close attention to the status of your hair system and the security of the bonding tapes or glues, and tend to the hair growth below the hair system.

Disguising the odor

Bacteria grow on the exfoliated skin and sebum (body oils) build up under hair replacement systems — an unpleasant thought, we know. It's only a matter of time until the smell of this bacterial growth begins to radiate from around your head. Regular hygiene is difficult with a hair system that has a more permanent type of attachment than one you can remove nightly.

You can combat bad smells by frequently washing your hair system. If you have two hair systems, you can remove one and replace it with the other while you wash and dry the first. However, washing a hair system causes progressive damage — the more it's washed, the quicker it wears out. Most attachment techniques are designed to allow you to loosen one edge of the system to wash under it, and then reattach the edge. Wearers who choose to have their pieces glued on for a month or longer must take great care to wash under them regularly.

Our best advice is to assume the hair system has a smell and to react accordingly with regular washing. Pouring a bottle of cologne over your head is not a viable substitute!

Maintaining a no-touch zone

This is a law that most hair system wearers live by. Most hair system wearers fear detection when there's the slightest intimacy or physical touching above the neck. Hugging a relative or date without letting them touch your head is awkward; it produces a no-touch zone that hinders intimacy with your nearest and dearest.

Adjusting to gray

When your natural hair starts to turn gray or salt and pepper, your must either alter or replace your hair system to blend in with the changes, or dye your natural hair to match the hair system. Replacing the hair system with gray or salt and pepper hair isn't a big problem because a system usually wears out in two to three years and must be replaced anyway.

If you decide to alter the hair system you have, you can have some gray hair put in when repairing the mesh and putting more hair into the hair system; this method allows you to gradually adjust to gray. But this gradual alteration can be expensive. The key is to keep the hair system naturally color-matched to your existing hair.

As most wearers own between two and four units, each must be color-matched as they're changed and washed, and that matching adds up financially.

Continuing regular haircuts

If you aren't completely bald, you can't just cover up what's left of your natural hair and forget about it. Hair beneath and around a hair system continues to grow, needs to be washed, and may need to be colored if you're trying to maintain your natural hair color.

One do-it-yourself solution is to shave your head, but that's not practical for most women or for men who want to use the hair they have left to augment or attach the hair system. (We discuss different types of attachments in Chapter 6.)

You can look, but you better not touch

We know of a patient who believed (but wasn't positive) that his long-term girlfriend didn't know about his hair system, and he was obsessed with keeping his no-touch zone intact to guarantee that any suspicions she may have had weren't confirmed. When she tried to touch his hair in intimate situations, he managed to keep her from it. However, he couldn't prevent a wind from coming up and blowing off his hairpiece as he and his girlfriend were walking on the Las Vegas strip.

When the patient's hair system blew off, he ran after it and ducked into a nearby store, leaving his girlfriend on the street. He reattached the hair system in the store bathroom and then took the next flight to Los Angeles for an emergency hair transplant, sending his girlfriend back home to Washington, D.C., by herself. Months later, he called us from home to say that he'd taken off his hairpiece and finally was going to experiment to see if his girlfriend could tell the difference. Minutes later, he called again to say that she'd immediately gone for his hair when he left his guard down, and although he was sick with fear, he allowed her to run her fingers through his hair. She admitted to suspecting that he had a hair system and was happy to feel his lovely, soft hair.

This patient told us that this was one of the most suspenseful and exciting experiences he'd had in years, and he felt that the decision to have a hair transplant was worth every penny. His no-touch zone was gone in an instant, and that feeling of his girlfriend running her fingers through his hair was indescribable. They were married within a year of his hair growth!

Eating into your expense account

People assume that hair systems are the least expensive alternative to hair loss. But many people find that the long-term costs involved with upkeep and replacement are a major disadvantage that they didn't plan for financially.

You may be able to find hair systems sold in mail-order catalogues or over the Internet for a few hundred dollars, but a good quality system can cost between $1,000 and $5,000. (Remember, the better quality the system, the harder it is to detect.) It's common to buy one or more identical spares at the same time so that you can wear one while the other gets cleaned or repaired as necessary. Continued maintenance costs, replacements costs as your hair thins, changes in texture and color, and the like can all become quite expensive. (See Chapter 6 for a typical budget from one of our patients.)

Chapter 17

Ten Reasons to Consider a Hair Transplant

Deciding whether a hair transplant is right for you is difficult. You may not only be dealing with your own feelings about it but also those of your family and friends. In this chapter, we give you ten good reasons why a hair transplant may be just what the doctor ordered for you.

Bald Isn't Making You Feel Beautiful

Some people hesitate to get a hair transplant because they think doing so makes them vain. But let's face it: Everyone wants to feel good about their appearance and goes to some lengths to feel better about how they look. Being told by family members, as some of my patients have been, that "being bald was good enough for Grandpa and should be good enough for you," isn't a good reason to dismiss a hair transplant if you think it's what's best for you.

A hair transplant isn't a sign of weakness or insecurity. In fact, a number of powerful, successful men have had hair transplants. For example, the president of South Korea, Lee Myung Bak, is widely rumored to have had a hair transplant, and former Pakistani Prime Minister Nawaz Sharif and Italian Prime Minister Silvio Berlusconi are among those who have taken steps to reclaim their hair.

And it's also true that many bald men are considered very attractive. Among them are actors Taye Diggs, Omar Epps, and Bruce Willis. But a surprising number of people have oddly shaped heads or scars, warts, lumps, or bumps on their heads that they would prefer cover with hair. It's a wonderful form of makeup to make your head look more like everyone else's.

You'd Like a More Symmetrical Face

Here's something you probably never knew (unless you were an art major in college): A so-called perfect face follows the rule of symmetry, which states that symmetrical portions of facial features equal attractiveness. In other words, a face that can be divided into equal thirds is an attractive face. Most people's faces don't conform exactly to the rule of thirds (⅓ from chin to nose, ⅓ from nose to the bridge between the eyes, and ⅓ from the bridge between the eyes to the hairline). Men rarely have those exact proportions, but in today's society, a handsome male face typically has a hairline that, in its distance from hollow at the upper point where your nose meets your forehead to the start of the hair, is equal to or less than the distance between the nose and the chin, never longer.

We measure these elements of the face on every patient coming through our office when we design a replacement hairline. The adult male hairline, which we call the *mature hairline,* has an equal distance between the chin to nose tip and the gully of the nose between the eyes to hairline. So that's the distance we aim to create in a mature male hairline reconstruction.

Our 100-percent rule for determining hairline location is based on forehead creases. Look in the mirror and lift your eyebrows as high as you can. You see wrinkles in the forehead that are created by a muscle that lies beneath the skin; hair never grows on the skin on top of this muscle (below that crease). In children and women, the location of the hairline is at the highest wrinkle. The mature male hairline sits ⅔ inch above the highest wrinkle. This space reflects the normal recession of the hairline in the non-balding male; if the hairline rises further than ⅔ inch, it's an indication of early genetic recession and the beginning of patterned balding.

If you look in the mirror and lift your eyebrows, the highest crease is where the hairline resided when a boy was 10 years old. If he wrinkled his brow, the hairline would hug his lower drawn-in hairline. The second line is the mature hairline that formed between ages 19 to 29. The shaded area above the second line shows hairline recession forming a pattern that reflects early balding. If this man lifted his eyebrows and creased his brow, the highest crease would appear at the point where the lowest hairline shows.

 When your hairline creeps upward, the proportions of your face change. Bringing your hair back down to where it belongs can keep your facial proportions in their proper balance, which is critical for a non-balding man's hairline reconstruction.

You Don't Want People Talking to Your Forehead

A common complaint of people with rising hairlines is that when they meet someone, the other person's eyes immediately look north. Lack of direct eye-to-eye contact is very disconcerting for even the most secure of people. A nice hairline avoids this uncomfortable problem by keeping the face framed and companions' eyes from wandering up.

Even with significant thinning on the top of your head or crown, your appearance doesn't really change until the hairline starts to go and you lose the upper aspect of the frame to your face. Framing is an important facet in art. For example, what good is a Picasso painting worth millions if it's not mounted and framed properly? A high-quality frame can make even an average Joe's painting look like expensive art. A face with a well-placed hairline brings out the best in facial features. When there's no upper hairline, the forehead seems to go on forever!

 When a hair transplant is done and the hairline isn't placed in the proper position, the forehead remains wide. We've seen skilled hair transplants in which the doctor has placed the hairline higher than where we define the mature male hairline. Even if the grafts aren't detectable, locating the hairline higher than where it belongs still draws the eye to the abnormally long forehead.

You Don't Want the Lifetime Cost of a Hair System

If you're trying to solve your hair problem and save money, you may think that it's cheaper to buy a toupee or other hair system rather than have a hair transplant. A hair system (toupee or wigs; see Chapters 6 and 7 for a full discussion of both) can seem inexpensive at first, but with the upkeep and maintenance, the life-time expense can far surpass that of any hair transplant surgery. Good quality hair systems range from $1,000 to $5,000 per year. We know of one typical patient who spent over $16,000 in the course of five years to purchase a hair system and maintain it! And the next five years will cost him the same amount without adjusting to inflation. Although a hair transplant is a one-time investment often comparable to or less than the five-year cost of a wig, a wig or a toupee needs costly maintenance — not such a great deal for you. Hair transplants are the better deal on the basis of just costs alone.

A number of years ago, I (Dr. Rassman) had a meeting with Sy Sperling, owner of Hair Club for Men, when he needed an affiliation with a doctor to go into the hair transplant business. At that time, he told me that the average income the company budgeted from a hair system over a five-year period was approximately $12,500. That was in 1996, so calculate what inflation has done to this cost! I doubt that the costs have come down.

A Bald Head Runs Hot and Cold

Hair is more than a vanity symbol; it keeps your head warm in the cold months of winter and protected from the sun in the heat of the summer. Hair works as a natural source of insulation — as any bald person can tell you. It has been calculated that people lose 50 percent of their body heat through the head when in freezing temperatures! Napoleon's army lost the bald men first in the freezing Russian winter. Although fighting in the Artic climes may not be in your future, a winter in a Northern climate can feel almost as cold at times.

In addition to the insulation it provides in cold weather, hair also provides cool shade when the weather is hot and the sun is strong, and it protects your scalp against the UV rays of the sun, keeping down the risk of skin cancer.

You're Tired of Toupees, Creams, and Other Disguises

As a bald man, what can you do about your condition? The non-surgical options are many, but they may all seem less than attractive. For example, grow a foot-long strand of hair to comb across the top, and you may be laughed out of town (see the section "You're Ready to Ditch the Infamous Comb-over" later in this section for more on this so-called solution to hair loss). Ditto for wearing inexpensive, obvious toupees, the worst of which give the impression of a small furry animal draped over the head. Much-hyped hair restoratives like Rogaine usually are only successful, if they are successful, on top-of-the-crown bald spots — if those spots haven't already expanded beyond the diameter of a small potato chip. Unfortunately, Rogaine doesn't grow back the hair to full thickness. You could shave your scalp, concealing your shame by pretending to revel in it. Or you can grow a beard to shift public attention to the nether end of your head. With all these proposed solutions, nobody has to suspect that you're actually bald, but they likely will anyway because non-surgical solutions are less effective at concealing hair loss than a hair transplant. Also, you're likely to get really sick of toupees, creams, and other disguises really fast.

You Want to Improve Your First Impression

No one likes to be judged by their appearance, but unfortunately, appearances do matter, and it's hard for people to get to know the real you if they can't get past the first impression. The reality is that the first impression is usually a physical one — whether it's in person or in a photo, such as on a dating Web site.

When it comes to dating, other things being equal, most men and women prefer a partner with a full head of hair because of a perception that balding reflects an older, less vibrant, and less sexually capable man. Hair has been unfairly, and incorrectly, associated with health and youth. Women see men with hair loss and automatically assume the men are unhealthy or old.

You're Ready to Go Au Naturel

"Au naturel," French for "in the natural (state)," is often used to mean "nude," but when it comes to hair, nude isn't always your best option! There's nothing wrong with having hair . . . up there! A hair transplant today looks and feels like your natural hair, growing like it did before it disappeared! You get a hair transplant and then forget about it except for routine haircuts. Wigs, toupees, and hats only offer a temporary cover up, whereas a hair transplant is a permanent and natural solution to baldness.

Many people have a negative opinion of hair transplants as looking unnatural. Terms such as "doll's head" or "plugs" come to mind. But today's hair transplant procedures have evolved. For example, follicular unit transplantation (FUT) is a technique in which hair is transplanted from the permanent zone in the back of the scalp into areas affected by genetic balding, using only the naturally occurring, individual follicular units. If performed well, the results are undetectable even to the trained eye. A good, modern hair transplant is undetectable to anyone not in the know about your original follicular state. The look is completely au naturel.

You're Ready to Ditch the Infamous Comb-over

In the beginning of our hair restoration practice, we couldn't help notice the most common hair style for balding men: the slicked side-to-side hair that runs from just above one ear to the other side over the bald head. The comb-over, as it's commonly known, has been popular with many men who grow the hair in the donor area (normally the sides/back of head for men) longer than normal to cover the balding area. Eventually, less and less hair is available to cover more and more surface area as the balding progresses.

We've always wondered how men reach the stage of the comb-over as a solution for their hair loss. It's clear that this style is a process that takes years to evolve as the man tries to preserve his old hair style by making use of ever diminishing quantities of hair. A comb-over style works for most men until the hair loss gets too bad and the bald area is too large. This is such a slow insidious process that most men don't notice it happening. John McCain is a good example of a man who uses the comb style and it is on the cusp of looking foolish.

How do the friends and families of these men with advanced, foolish-looking comb-overs keep their mouths shut about how silly it looks? It seems that they just go along with the deception to protect their loved one's feelings, or they may be just too embarrassed to speak the truth. If you love someone, you can usually manage to overlook their imperfections, if not downright oddities, but the staring eyes from friends and strangers can sometimes be a bit much to bear. When you reach a point at which you're ready to ditch your comb-over, a hair transplant is the best next step you can take.

You Don't Like Using Sun Screen on Your Head

The presence of a bald crown or a bald head produces a problem that most non-bald men never think about. Sun burns! And these sun burns eventually lead to a type of skin cancer. If you look carefully at the head of a balding man over the age of 50 or so, you will see darkened spots on the bald areas of the scalp. Many of these spots are precancerous lesions and they must be checked frequently by a good dermatologist.

Chapter 18

Ten Facts about the FDA and Hair Products

*I*n the United States, it's common to assume that the U.S. Food and Drug Administration (FDA) looks out for consumer's welfare when it comes to hair products, from over-the-counter drugs to medical devices for stimulating hair growth.

But does it? As this chapter reveals, the answer is both yes and no.

If you're wondering what the FDA's mission is, here is its mission statement:

> The FDA is responsible for protecting the public health by assuring the safety, efficacy, and security of human and veterinary drugs, biological products, medical devices, our nation's food supply, cosmetics, and products that emit radiation. The FDA is also responsible for advancing the public health by helping to speed innovations that make medicines and foods more effective, safer, and more affordable; and helping the public get the accurate, science-based information they need to use medicines and foods to improve their health.

Sounds like some lofty goals and really big jobs, and they are. But, not too surprisingly, the FDA can't be everywhere all the time, which is why contaminated medications, tainted food, and dangerous devices *do* occasionally make it onto the market. However, the FDA does its best to keep things safe.

What is the FDA's involvement in hair loss issues? Well, snake oil salesmen and charlatans still have no trouble pedaling their products to hairless and desperate consumers. In this chapter, we look at the myths and truths about what the FDA does and doesn't do when it comes to hair loss.

It Doesn't Approve Shampoos and Conditioners

Yes, it's true — the FDA wants you and your dermatologist to know what's in your shampoo and conditioner and mandates that shampoo and conditioner manufacturers list all ingredients on the backs of the containers. The agency also prohibits manufacturers from making any false claims about what your shampoo or conditioner can do for your hair.

Most shampoos and conditioners are regulated as *cosmetics,* which means that companies can put them on the market without prior FDA approval. This fast-track to store shelves doesn't mean cosmetics are unsafe. In fact, most shampoos and hair conditioners are perfectly safe when used as directed. Care should be taken to keep shampoos out of the eyes because that, as you know, can cause stinging. Some consumers who use the same shampoo for years can develop an allergy to it and should switch to another brand.

However, not all shampoos and conditioners are created equal. Shampoos that contain ingredients designed to treat conditions such as dandruff or psoriasis are regulated by the FDA as *drugs*, not cosmetics, and that means those shampoos are subject to more extensive regulations, as discussed later in this chapter.

It Doesn't Approve Most Permanent Hair Dyes

As we explain in Chapter 3, there are three types of hair dye:

- ✔ Permanent
- ✔ Semi-permanent
- ✔ Temporary

All three types can contain *coal-tar dyes,* potent chemicals that can cause potential safety problems, including irritation and allergy. Note that "Coal-tar" dyes are not really made from coal-tar anymore. They are made from petroleum but the old name is still found in FDA regulations and FDA laws.

One type of permanent hair dye is the "progressive" type. This dye contains either lead acetate or bismuth citrate, both of which have been approved and listed in the Code of Federal Regulations for coloring scalp hair only as a result of petitions submitted to the FDA. Henna has also been listed.

Unlike color additives used in other cosmetic products, Congress exempted oxidation-type coal-tar hair dyes from its listing and certification regulations. In such cases, all the agency can do is require adequate directions for preliminary patch testing by consumers for skin sensitivity and that the following warning statement appear on the label:

> Caution: This product contains ingredients which may cause skin irritation on certain individuals and a preliminary test according to accompanying directions should first be made. This product must not be used for dyeing the eyelashes or eyebrows; to do so may cause blindness.

Since anyone can become sensitized to hair dyes with time, patch tests are urged each time before a consumer intends to use an oxidation hair dye.

Oxidation (or "coal-tar") hair dyes contain synthetic organic dyes and dye intermediates made from petroleum that penetrate the hair shaft in the presence of hydrogen peroxide and ammonia. This results in a coloring of the hair that lasts a long time.

A few permanent dyes have been shown to cause cancer in animals.

Progressive hair dyes are made with lead acetate, or less frequently, bismuth citrate. These FDA-approved dyes gradually darken the hair by oxidizing on the hair surface and reacting with the sulfur in the keratin of the hair shaft. (Refer to Chapter 2 for an explanation of the structure of hair.)

Semi-permanent and temporary dyes also contain coal-tar dyes, but they adhere to the surface of the hair shaft for much shorter periods of time than permanent dyes.

FDA Gets Help from the Courts to Protect Consumers

It's no surprise that the FDA gets the most complaints from consumers about hair relaxers (straighteners) and hair dyes. Each contain powerful chemicals that can cause harm, especially if used incorrectly by consumers that do not understand the risks.

The FDA tries to inform the consumers to take a proactive approach in using such products safely. The agency also reviews consumer complaints and, when it finds a pattern of unusual or severe reactions, it conducts an investigation and requests a company to voluntarily remove the product from the market. But the agency doesn't have pre-approval authority for cosmetics and sometimes needs help in getting an unsafe product off the market.

Take the example of the World Rio Corporation of California. It marketed two hair relaxers, the Rio Naturalizer System (Neutral Formula) and the Rio Naturalizer System with Color Enhancer (Black/Licorice). Consumers had complained to the FDA about hair loss, scalp irritation, and discolored hair. The FDA requested that the company cease marketing these products. In December 1994, they agreed to stop sales and shipments of the products.

The FDA discovered, however, that the company had continued to take orders. The California Department of Health then also asked them to stop sales. Finally, in January 1995, the U.S. Attorney's Office in Los Angeles filed a seizure action against these products on behalf of the FDA.

In the resulting consent decree of condemnation and permanent injunction, the FDA noted that it received more than 3,000 complaints about the Rio products. The agency alleged that the products were potentially harmful or injurious when used as intended, that they were more acidic than declared in the labeling, and that the labeling described the products as "chemical free" when "allegedly they contained ingredients commonly understood to be 'chemicals.'"

Hair relaxers (known also as hair straighteners) are generally alkaline rather than acidic products. Lye or another strongly alkaline chemical is used to break the bonds in the hair. Lye can cause burns to the scalp if left on too long or not properly washed out with shampoo and conditioner. Getting help from someone else in applying and removing the relaxer can help ensure all is removed and neutralized.

Since lye can cause burns to the face, lungs, and esophagus if swallowed, parents are urged to keep this product out of reach of children. When using a relaxer on children, be especially careful to keep it off the skin and out of their eyes.

Since hair relaxers can result in hair breakage, baldness, burns, and emergency room visits, special care is urged when using these products. Some people use petroleum jelly on their heads to form a protective barrier before using a hair relaxer. A neutralizing shampoo should be used after treatment, followed by a hair conditioner. Consumers should avoid scratching their heads or brushing hair before using a relaxer.

And don't leave the relaxer on too long! Using a relaxer too frequently can damage the hair. It's also not a good idea to use a permanent oxidation (coal tar) dye the same day as you use a hair relaxer because the chance of hair damage increases.

It Protects You from Cosmetic Hair Growth Product Scams

In 1989, the FDA, concerned about consumer gullibility, banned all topical lotions, potions, creams, and other cosmetic gunk that claimed to grow hair where there was no hair. However, these products have now begun to crop up on the Internet. From the FDA's perspective, shutting down these scams must be like picking fleas off a dog — every time they remove one, another one jumps up.

The bottom line? No matter what you see and hear on late-night TV, a product can't grow a single hair on your head if you have nothing to start with. You can write to the FDA or Federal Trade Commission (FTC) to complain about such products. The FDA regulates labeling claims while the FTC regulates advertising.

It Approves All Prescription Drugs That Claim to Grow Hair

You can rest assured that any new prescription drug claiming to grow new hair has been thoroughly tested in clinical trials. After a certain number of years, though, the patent on brand name drugs expires, and other companies can manufacture the same drug under a different name as a generic drug.

For example, under the brand name Proscar, finasteride was manufactured by Merck and originally covered by U.S. and international patents to treat benign prostate hypertrophy (BPH). A separate patent for the drug was issued to treat male pattern baldness under the name Propecia.

Finasteride is now off-patent for use in treating BPH and is sold under several generic names. Propecia won't be off-patent until 2013, at which time generic versions will undoubtedly appear.

Because generic drug makers don't develop a drug from scratch, their costs to bring the drug to market are much lower, but they must show that their product works in the same way as the brand-name drug. No clinical trials, however, are required. All generic drugs are approved by the FDA, and the FDA assures the public that they're equivalent to the original medications.

It Doesn't Pre-Approve Over-the-Counter Hair Growth Drugs

Drugs that are sold over-the-counter (OTC) aren't subject to pre-market FDA approval, but it does oversee OTC drugs to ensure that they're properly labeled and that their benefits outweigh their risks. There are more than 80 classes of OTC drugs, including products for hair growth and loss, antifungal products, sunscreen, and weight-control drugs.

Particular classes of OTC drugs are subject to a *monograph* system. *Monographs* specify the active ingredients, labeling, and testing required for the particular class of drugs. For example, if you want to market a sunscreen, you can follow the sunscreen monograph and go to market without submitting anything to the FDA (except manufacturer registration and drug listing information). However, if you want to add substantial new claims to a new sunscreen or change the percentages of active ingredients that appear in the monograph, you need to submit a very expensive new drug application for FDA approval. The monograph system is a convenient one for most manufacturers, but it does inhibit development of improved products.

The FDA published a report in 1989, the *Final Monograph on Hair Grower and Hair Loss-Prevention OTC Drug Products for Human Use,* after a review of safety and efficacy data submitted by interested companies. The FDA was, to say the least, unimpressed with what it received, and the Monograph stated, "There are no agency-approved OTC hair loss prevention drug products" and warned companies not to market such products unless they want to risk FDA action.

That's why you don't see OTC drugs with hair loss prevention claims in your pharmacy.

It Prevents Dietary Supplements from Claiming to Cure Hair Loss

A *dietary supplement* is defined as "a product taken by mouth that contains a 'dietary ingredient' intended to supplement the diet." Dietary supplements can be extracts or concentrates and may be found in many forms, such as tablets, capsules, softgels, gelcaps, liquids, or powders.

Manufacturers of dietary supplements usually don't need to register their products with the FDA and generally don't need FDA approval before producing or selling dietary supplements. The Dietary Supplement Health and Education Act (DSHEA) instituted in 1994 says that the FDA is only responsible for taking action against an unsafe dietary supplement after it's on the market.

It's illegal to market a dietary supplement product as a treatment or cure for a specific disease or condition, such as hair loss. Many supplements and herbal remedies are nevertheless illegally advertised as being able to cure hair loss. If you see a topical dietary supplement with such claims, you can be sure that it's illegal.

Advertising claims are regulated not by the FDA but by the Federal Trade Commission (FTC). When a product has been proven unsafe, such as what happened with Ephedra, the FDA can order it removed from the market. But before that point, it's up to you to be a careful and sensible consumer when buying supplements.

It Doesn't Require Much from Class 1 Medical Devices

Medical devices fall into one of three classes with increasing complexity and potential risk. *Class I devices* aren't intended for use in supporting or sustaining life or to be of substantial importance in preventing impairment to human health. They also can't present a potential unreasonable risk of illness or injury.

Medical devices are usually exempt from premarket notification submission requirements (the 510(k), a lower standard than FDA approval that comes from an abbreviated process). The author (Dr. Rassman) produced a medical instrument, 'the hair implanter pen (HIP)' and this is an example of such a class I cleared device.

It Requires Clearance for Class II Medical Devices

Class II devices, including those for hair growth, require special labeling and are held to a higher standard than Class I devices; sponsors of the 510(k) must show the FDA that the proposed device is at least as safe and effective as similar legally marketed products in the U.S. Devices in this class are typically noninvasive and include products like low-level laser therapy devices that claim to grow new hair (http://en.wikipedia.org/wiki/Medical_device - endnote_FDA3132). Most Class II products require 510(k) clearance, which is a lower standard than FDA approval.

One device that went through the 510(k) process and is now touted on many Web sites as "FDA approved" is the low-level laser treatment for home use, called the HairMax LaserComb(r). The sponsor made the medical claim that this medical device could grow hair, and that claim had to be addressed by the FDA before the product could go on the market.

Because the LaserComb is a Class II product, the company only had to show that it was as safe and effective as similar legally marketed U.S. products. Only one study was done to show that the LaserComb was safe and effective before it was cleared for marketing.

It Requires Thorough Testing and Trials for Class III Devices

Class III medical devices need to be thoroughly tested in clinical trials to ensure their safety and effectiveness over and above the Class I and Class II controls. Examples include coronary heart valves and stents. Hair care products and devices don't fall into the Class III category unless someone invents something that's life-supporting or life-sustaining and also grows hair.

Currently, with one exception, the hair-growing tools sold in your local drugstore or big box store aren't likely to be FDA approved or even to have FDA clearance because their claims are limited and their risks are low.

Part VII
Appendixes

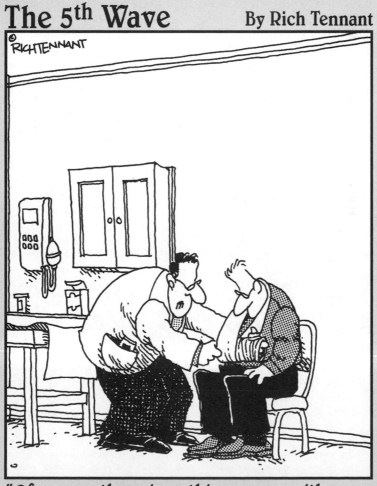

The 5th Wave   By Rich Tennant

"Of course there is nothing wrong with your arm, but it will keep people from focusing on your hair transplant."

In this part . . .

This part contains three appendixes. The first collection of professional associations and Internet resources relating to hair loss. The second summarizes the results a study we did about the psychological changes in men who had hair transplants. Considering a hair transplant and wondering if it will be worth it, psychologically speaking? This appendix will give you valuable information gleaned from men who've been through the process.

Finally we have included the a glossary to help you identify scientific or unfamiliar terms used in this book, since this book, like any medically oriented book, contains some technical jargon.

Appendix A

Online Organizations and Resources

● ●

*I*nformation on hair loss is everywhere, if you know where to look. The following resources direct you to organizations and Web sites that can help you stay current on information relating to hair loss and treatments.

Dr. Rassman's Web Sites and Blogs

True, I'm a bit biased, but I think these Web sites are comprehensive references that provide a truly educational resource for understanding hair loss and the latest medical and surgical treatments of baldness. And because they're my personal Web sites, I naturally think they're among the best!

- ✔ **New Hair Institute** (www.newhair.com)
- ✔ **Bernstein Medical** (www.bernsteinmedical.com)
- ✔ **Balding Blog** (www.baldingblog.com)
- ✔ **Hair Transplant Blog** (www.bernsteinmedical.com/hairtransplantblog)

These sites offer detailed explanations to the most commonly asked questions about hair loss and provide an in-depth resource for information on more detailed issues relating to hair restoration surgery. With photos, diagrams, video, and useful links, these sites offer a virtual encyclopedia for the treatment of hair loss. As of this writing, BaldingBlog.com alone features more than 6,000 entries. Feel free to write to me.

Other Web Sites Devoted to Hair Loss

A number of Web sites provide information, discussion forums, and question-and-answer formats. Here are some places to start.

- ✔ **Alopecia Areata Support Group** (www.mdjunction.com): This site is a meeting place for people who want to connect with others dealing with the same hair disease challenges as they are.

- ✔ **National Alopecia Areata Foundation** (www.naaf.org): This resource is a thorough collection of articles, pictures, and comprehensive material related to Alopecia Areata.

- ✔ **The Bald Truth** (www.thebaldtruth.com): This hair loss consumer resource includes recommended hair loss products, discussion forums, chat, news, and much more.

- ✔ **Hair Loss Help** (hairlosshelp.com): A good source of information on hair loss treatments. The site has forums and chats on hair loss therapies and information on the drugs Rogaine and Propecia as well as other medications, hair loss research, natural treatments, and cosmetic cover-ups.

- ✔ **Hair Transplant Network** (www.hairtransplantnetwork.com): This site helps hair loss sufferers share ideas and experiences about treatments and hair restoration physicians. This popular online community includes hundreds of patient photos, recommendations for over 50 of the world's leading hair restoration physicians, and a popular hair loss discussion forum.

- ✔ **Hair Doctor Guide** (www.hairdoctorguide.com): This site contains a list of doctors who have solid reputations in the hair field as well as those who have a particular interest in either medical and/or surgical treatment for hair loss and hair diseases. It also lists a variety of bulletin boards, hair transplant communities, and discussion groups that may not have been available when this book was first printed and where patients or patient advocates can share their experiences and knowledge. This site will be regularly updated and dynamic, so at the time of the printing of this book, this site will be under construction.

- ✔ **Hair Loss Advisor** (www.hairlossadvisor.com): An online source of information about hair loss prevention and treatment delivering streaming-media-based events with healthcare professionals.

General Medical Web Sites

These Web sites are devoted to a number of health issues but do contain articles related to hair loss.

- ✔ **Castle Connolly** (www.castleconnolly.com): Castle Connolly Medical Ltd. is a research and information company founded in 1992 to help consumers find top doctors and top hospitals. Find detailed information about education, training, and special expertise of America's best doctors.

- ✔ **CNN Health** (www.cnn.com/health): This site is among the world's leaders in online medical news and information, providing live video and audio streaming and searchable archives of health features and background information.

- ✔ **Derm Atlas** (www.dermatlas.org): Dermatology image atlas with over 7,000 dermatologic images collected and edited by Johns Hopkins dermatologists. It was originally created for health care professionals, including dermatology residents and dermatologists.

- ✔ **Discovery Health** (health.discovery.com): Created by the Discovery Channel, this site provides resources and stories on important health issues including baldness.

- ✔ **eMedicine** (www.emedicine.com): Includes more than 5,500 pages of health content, written by physicians for patients and consumers. Each article is reviewed by a panel of physicians. Current medical information includes good overviews of causes and treatments for hair loss.

- ✔ **Health On the Net Foundation** (www.hon.ch/): This site is a non-governmental organization whose mission is to guide lay persons or non-medical users and medical practitioners to useful and reliable online medical and health information.

- ✔ **The National Library of Medicine** (www.nlm.nih.gov/): This resource is the world's largest medical library. The library collects materials in all areas of biomedicine and health care, as well as works on biomedical aspects of technology; the humanities; and the physical, life, and social sciences. The collections stand at more than 7 million items — books, journals, technical reports, manuscripts, microfilms, photographs, and images.

- ✔ **Web MD** (www.webmd.com): Provides expertise in medicine, journalism, health communication, and content creation to bring health information, tools for managing health, and support to those who seek information.

Sites that Contain Specific Drug Info

The following sites contain information aimed at professionals and laymen on drugs related to hair loss.

✔ **Follicle** (www.follicle.com): This site provides detailed information on alopecia specifically as related to the drug Propecia.

✔ **Propecia** (www.propecia.com): This is the official site for Propecia, the first and only FDA-approved pill demonstrated to treat male pattern hair loss on the vertex and anterior mid-scalp area in men only.

✔ **Rogaine** (www.rogaine.com): This site is your official source for info on Rogaine, the brand name for minoxidil. The solution is applied to the scalp daily to stimulate hair growth and help prevent hair loss. It's available over-the-counter in the U.S.

Sites with Specific Product Info

The following sites provide information of products used to cover hair loss.

✔ **Hair Outlet Store** (www.hairoutletstore.com): A listing of various hair products researched by Dr. Rassman as well as a listing of ingredients found in those products. This site will be regularly updated and dynamic so at the time of the printing of this book, this site will be under construction.

✔ **Couvre** (www.toppik.com/couvre.asp): A cream that darkens the scalp to match the hair; you dab it on with your fingers. It's made of a sesame seed emulsion that isn't greasy or sticky and doesn't rub off or stain. It doesn't come off when you're exercising, perspiring, or even swimming, but you can easily remove it with shampooing.

Contact Spencer Forest Labs, 64 Post Road West, Westport, CT 06880.

✔ **DermMatch** (www.dermatch.com): DermMatch is a hard-packed powdered cosmetic you apply with a wet sponge applicator. It coats thin hairs to make them thicker and helps them stand up and spread out for increased fullness. Plus, it conditions your hair and moisturizes your skin. DermMatch also colors your skin to match your hair color, causing the scalp to disappear, and it's the only product you can fade to mimic a hairline. You're able to brush your hair and swim with it. You apply it with a wet sponge applicator.

Contact DermMatch, Inc., 777 Shamrock Blvd., Venice, FL 34293; Phone: 800-826-2824.

✔ **Fullmore** (www.toppik.com/fullmore.asp): Fullmore is a colored hair-thickening spray that makes your hair look naturally thicker and fuller in seconds by covering thinning areas and adding texture and volume to thinning hair. It has an easy spray-on applicator.

Contact Spencer Forest Labs, 64 Post Road West, Westport, CT 06880Phone: 800-416-3325.

✔ **ProTHIK** (www.prothik.com/index.htm): ProTHIK is an aerosol hair thickening spray-on system that cosmetically eliminates bald spots in the *vertex* (crown) or other localized thinning areas. It contains a thickening resin that is rub- and water-resistant.

Contact ProTHIK at 800-710-8445.

✔ **Toppik** (www.toppik.com/toppik.asp): Toppik is a complex of tiny, microfiber hairs that blend with your own hair. Toppik fibers, derived from the keratin in wool, are made of the same organic keratin protein as your own hair. The fibers change thin, fine hair into hair that appears thicker and fuller. You apply Toppik by gently shaking the custom container over thinning area. In this process, thousands of tiny color-matched hair fibers intertwine with your own hair. Charged with static electricity, they bond so that they stay in place for hours. Toppik comes in eight different colors.

Contact Spencer Forest Labs, 64 Post Road West, Westport, CT 06880; Phone: 800-416-3325.

Professional Web Sites and Journals

These sources of information for professionals can keep you up to date on the latest in hair replacement, if you can manage to wade through the medical terminology.

✔ **Archives of Dermatology** (www.archderm.ama-assn.org): This site publishes information concerning the skin, its diseases, and their treatment. Its mission is to fully explain the structure and function of the skin and its diseases and the art of using this information to deliver optimal medical and surgical care to the patient.

✔ **Cutis** (www.cutis.com): This publication is a 40-year-old, peer-reviewed clinical journal for the dermatologist, allergist, and general practitioner. The journal comes out monthly and focuses on concise clinical articles that present the practical side of dermatology.

✔ **Dermatologic Surgery** (mc.manuscriptcentral.com/ds): This journal publishes peer-reviewed articles on all aspects of dermatologic surgery and oncology, including clinical studies, surgical procedures, review articles, and experimental studies.

✔ **National Library of Medicine** (www.nlm.nih.org): On the campus of the National Institutes of Health in Bethesda, Maryland, is the world's largest medical library. The library collects materials and provides information and research services in all areas of biomedicine and health care.

✔ **New England Journal of Medicine** (www.content.nejm.org): This publication is a weekly general medical journal that publishes new medical research findings, review articles, and editorial opinion on a wide variety of topics of importance to biomedical science and clinical practice.

Professional Organizations

These sources can help you find a doctor you can trust.

✔ **The American Academy of Cosmetic Surgery (AACS)** (www.cosmeticsurgery.org): This group is the largest affiliation of doctors who have training in cosmetic surgery. It's a not-for-profit organization providing information on cosmetic surgery for patients, physicians, and the media. The site includes a physician search and procedural information.

✔ **The American Academy of Dermatology (AAD)** (www.aad.org): This group is the largest, most influential and most representative of all dermatologic associations. With a membership of over 13,700, it represents virtually all practicing dermatologists in the United States.

✔ **American Board of Dermatology (ABD)** (www.abderm.org): The ABD acts as the certifying agency for the specialty of dermatology. It exists for the primary purpose of protecting the public interest by establishing and maintaining high standards of training, education, and qualifications of physicians rendering care in dermatology.

✔ **American Board of Hair Restoration Surgery (ABHRS)** (www.abhrs.com): ABHRS acts for the benefit of the public to establish specialty standards and to examine surgeons' skill, knowledge, and aesthetic judgment in the field of hair restoration surgery.

✔ **American Medical Association (AMA)** (www.ama-assn.org): This association is the nation's largest physicians group advocating vital national health issues.

✔ **American Society for Dermatologic Surgery (ASDS)** (www.asds.net): ASDS was founded in 1970 to promote excellence in the subspecialty of dermatologic surgery and foster the highest standards of patient care.

✔ **American Society of Plastic Surgeons (ASPS)** (www.plasticsurgery.org): This group is the largest plastic surgery specialty organization in the world. Founded in 1931, the society is composed of board-certified plastic surgeons that perform cosmetic and reconstructive surgery.

Appendix B

A Psychological Study of Hair Loss

● ●

C linicians who work in the field of hair loss, as we do, know full well that hair loss has a psychological impact on many aspects of a person's life. We see patients every day whose lives have changed for the better after transplant, and it's well established that men and women with depression are more likely to be bald than not.

We decided to send out a questionnaire asking about the psychological impact of hair loss and hair transplantation to 200 hair transplant clients. A study looking at the benefits of hair transplantation on psychological issues such as stress levels and self-esteem had never been done before. This appendix explains what we learned.

The research was conducted at the New Hair Institute by Parsa Mohebi, M.D., and William R. Rassman, M.D.

What the Survey Asked

Our survey focused on the following seven variables:

- ✔ General level of happiness
- ✔ Energy level
- ✔ Feeling of youthfulness
- ✔ Anxiety level
- ✔ Self-confidence
- ✔ Outlook on the future
- ✔ Impact on sex life

The survey asked patients to rate their psychological states before and after hair transplant surgery.

Who Was Surveyed

We mailed our survey to patients who fit the following categories:

- Male patients with male pattern baldness
- Patients whose surgeries had been done in the past 1 to 3 years, so that the memory of their lives before transplant were still fresh in their minds
- Patients who had had only one transplant
- Patients who had the follicular unit transplant

We sent the survey with a brief explanation of what we hoped to accomplish (and a self-addressed stamped envelope). The questionnaire was *blind,* meaning it contained no client identifiers of any kind. Individuals didn't have cause to worry that we would know who they were. Participation was completely voluntary, and no incentives of any kind were given for participating.

What the Survey Showed

We received 37 questionnaires back from our survey, for an 18.5 percent return rate. The most immediate and striking result was that *all* patients showed significant improvements in *all* eight areas. The results are shown in Figure B-1.

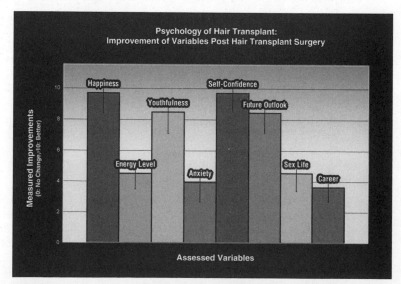

Figure B-1: Comparison of psychological variables before and after hair transplant.

Comparing older and younger patients

We broke the results down by age, dividing patients into under and over age 40 groups to see if there were any differences between the two groups. The results are shown in Figure B-2.

Younger patients, perhaps not unexpectedly, felt that their transplant had a larger impact on their future than older patients did. Patients who experienced hair loss at an earlier age, while involved in an active social life, experienced more negative effects from balding and benefited the most from hair transplantation.

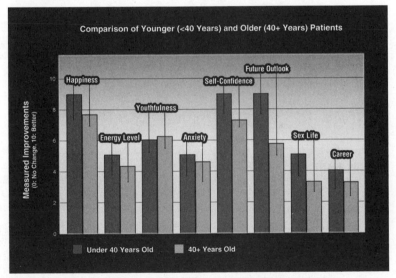

Figure B-2: Comparison of younger patients to older patients.

Comparing different balding patterns

We took the resulting data a step further to see if the type of balding pattern a patient had made any difference in his final results. We broke the group into two: one group with Norwood pattern III-IV (low hair loss), and the other group with Norwood pattern V-VII (high class of hair loss). (See Chapter 4 for more on the Norwood classifications in hair loss.) See Figure B-3.

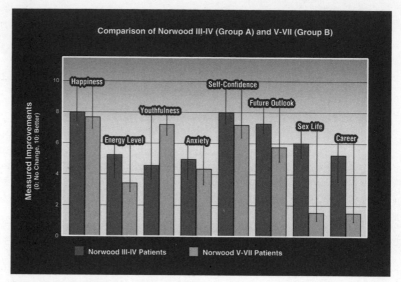

Figure B-3: Comparison of patients with low Norwood classification to those with higher classification.

Analyzing the Results

This study confirmed what we already knew from talking to patients: Hair loss causes or worsens psychological problems such as anxiety, fear in social situations, and even difficulties in career advancement.

The good news is that reversing hair loss, particularly in younger men who have less balding at the time of transplant, can reverse its negative psychological effects and increase psychological satisfaction in many life situations.

Although this study was valuable, our goal is to do a much larger study. It's admittedly difficult to get people to respond to a blind survey without some type of incentive, so a larger, funded study may result in more data.

Many people continue to feel that hair loss is nothing more than a vanity issue and that concern about it is unwarranted. This study, however, shows very clearly that hair loss is more than a vanity issue; it has a profound effect on every aspect of a person's life.

The research was conducted by Parsa Mohebi, M.D. and William Rassman, M.D.

Appendix C

Glossary

• •

*L*ike many technical and medical topics, hair loss comes with its own set of terminology. This glossary is designed to simplify your reading and understanding of this book by giving you one source for definitions related to hair and hair loss.

alopecia: The medical term for genetic hair loss.

alopecia areata (AA): A type of inherited skin disease that produces hair loss. AA often begins as patches of hair loss that spread into larger and larger areas.

anabolic steroids: A group of hormones made from testosterone that promotes tissue growth and the building of proteins.

anagen phase: The phase of the hair cycle when hair is growing. The anagen phase lasts from between from one to seven years with an average length of three years.

androgenic (or androgenetic) alopecia: Hair loss caused by a combination of the male hormone and genes; also known as male pattern baldness.

anti-androgen: Any substance that suppresses the production or the effects of the male hormone testosterone.

apoptosis: A genetic process that produces cell destruction, failure to grow, or cell death. Genes determine how many hair cycles a particular hair will go through. The mechanism of how this works probably relates to particular growth-stimulating molecules that must be present for a hair to grow out. The genetic determination of how many cycles a hair will go through and when that number is reached occurs because some critical molecule fails to be produced. Each individual hair has a different cycle, so the death of any particular hair varies by regions on the scalp and the genes that are inherited from one's parents.

aromatase: An enzyme that facilitates the conversion of the male hormone testosterone into the female hormone estrogen. A healthy hair is hormone dependent, and that dependency requires the presence of both male and female hormones in some balance. In women, a deficiency of aromatase causes an estrogen deficiency, and estrogen supports healthy hair growth. When estrogen levels are low in women, they experience hair loss, which explains why so many women have hair loss when they go through menopause.

autosomal gene: A gene found on the non-sex chromosome.

catagen phase: The phase of the hair cycle during which the hair prepares for its sleep phase and falls out.

chromophore: A molecule that absorbs light waves at a specific wavelength and imparts a color to the molecule. Two types of pig-ment molecules (called *melanin*) are produced at the base of the hair bulb: eumelanin and phaeomelanin. All hair colors result from a balance between these two molecules. See *eumelanin* and *phaeomelanin.*

cobblestoning: Changes in the skin that appear like a cobblestone street surface. The large plug hair transplants performed prior to 1990 produced such changes on the bald scalp.

cortex: The inner layer of a hair shaft found inside the cuticle. The cortex contains bundles of compressed protein that make up the inner part of the hair shaft.

cuticle: The outermost layer of a hair shaft. The cuticle is porous and made up of scales, and it surrounds the inner elements that make up the hair shaft.

cysteine: An amino acid readily oxidized to cystine.

cyproterone acetate: An anti-androgen that suppresses the action of testosterone.

hydroepiandrosterone (DHEA): A weak steroid secreted by the adrenal gland. As an androgenic steroid, it can cause hair loss. Some people take this as a supplement and may very well increase their hair loss. The mechanism of its action appears to be in the metabolism of DHEA, which produces DHT (dihydrotestosterone), the hormone in men that causes hair loss.

dermal papillae: An area of the hair follicle located at the base of the hair bulb that's active in controlling the growth of the hair follicle.

dihydrotestosterone (DHT): A hormone made from testosterone and mediated by the enzyme 5-a reductase. This is the hormone responsible for secondary sex characteristics like body hair, beard hair, and changes in the voices of adolescent boys. DHT is also the hormone that causes hair loss when a man carries the genetics for hair loss.

diffuse unpatterned alopecia (DUPA): A disease of hair loss in which the entire scalp is impacted by microscopic miniaturization and visible thinning.

disulfide bonds: Part of the protein inside the cortex of the hair shaft that isn't water soluble and accounts for the strength of the protein making up the bundles of hair.

dominant gene: A gene found on a chromosome that's strongest and expresses itself in a dominant position over other similar genes.

dutasteride: An FDA-approved drug for the treatment of prostate enlargement that is presently under FDA consideration for the treatment of hair loss.

eumelanin: Pigment molecule that controls black and brown hair colors (produced by a dominant gene) and makes black or brown hair. Blonde hair occurs when the concentration of this eumelanin molecule is very low.

finasteride: An FDA-approved drug for the treatment of prostate enlargement and hair loss.

5-a reductase: An enzyme critical for the chemical breakdown of testosterone in producing dihydrotestosterone (DHT).

follicular unit: The basic hair follicular anatomy that contains between one and five hairs, blood vessels, nerves, and connective tissue.

follicular unit extraction: A minimally invasive surgery for removing follicular units for hair transplantation.

frontal fibrosing alopecia: A condition that causes hair loss and scarring in the frontal area of the scalp. It's most commonly found in women over age 50 and is thought to be an autoimmune disease.

hair follicle: A single hair and its production anatomy below the skin.

hair replacement system: An appliance containing hair that's worn on the head (also known as a "wig," "toupee," "hair piece," or "piece").

hair shaft: The hard, dead output of a follicular unit. The shaft is the part of the hair that shows above the skin and that is styled.

hair transplant: A surgical procedure in which hair is moved from one part of the body to another.

hydrogen bonds: Proteins inside the cortex of the hair shaft that are water soluble. These bonds break down easily and give hair its flexibility. Hydrogen bonds come apart when the hair is wet and come back together again as the hair dries.

laser: A device that stimulates a beam of coherent light. Some people believe that a laser imparts energy to the scalp and hair follicles and that this energy results in a positive impact on the growth of the hair. Unfortunately, the scientific proof for this theory is scant.

male pattern baldness: See *androgenic (or androgenetic) alopecia.*

medulla: An area of the hair shaft within the cortex.

megasession: A hair transplant session in which more than 1,000 follicular grafts are transplanted in a single session.

methionine: An amino acid containing sulfur, which is critical to the growth of healthy hair. A deficiency of sulfur can cause hair loss or weak hair. Sulfur is also critical in the production of healthy fingernails and toenails and is found all over the body, including the skin.

micrograft: A unit of hair containing between one and three hairs.

miniaturization: The process whereby the hair shafts on the scalp have a reduced diameter when compared with normal healthy hairs.

Minoxidil: A drug originally developed to treat high blood pressure but that's now used to treat hair loss topically.

Norwood classification: A classification of hair loss patterns as seen in men.

phaeomelanin: Pigment molecule that produces red tint in hair.

saw palmetto: An extract of the fruit Serenoa repens. It's sold in health food stores for medicinal value and is thought to have value in treating hair loss.

shock loss: Hair loss induced by some stressful event, such as hair transplant surgery.

single strip harvesting: The removal of a section of scalp by excision for the purpose of hair transplantation. The hair follicles in that section of scalp are removed from the scalp and inserted into the bald scalp at the recipient area.

spironolactone: A drug that's a weak diuretic and that has anti-androgen (male hormone) effects. Because of the anti-androgenic actions of this drug, doctors have been using it for years in the treatment of female hair loss. No reputable scientific studies show that it produces dependable, replicable results for hair growth.

telogen effluvium: A state of health in which many hair follicles on the scalp go into the hair cycle of sleep at the same time. This cycle lasts longer than the normal cycle length.

telogen phase: A phase of the hair cycle in which the hair enters a sleep phase. This phase lasts around 100 days on average.

testosterone: The male hormone produced by the testicles that's responsible for the male sex drive. This hormone is metabolized into DHT (dihydrotestosterone), which is the cause for hair loss in men with the genetic tendency for male pattern balding.

terminal hair: A fully grown hair that has normal thickness.

tinea capitus: A fungal disease of the hair and scalp that often causes hair loss. It's most frequently found in children and appears as patchy hair loss.

traction alopecia: Hair loss from constant pulling of hair. It often occurs as a result of styling or rubbing of the scalp. This process is often permanent.

transection: The process whereby the deep hair follicle below the skin is damaged or cut through. This occurs during the harvesting process of a hair transplant.

trichotillomania: A medical condition in which a person picks at his or her hair, causing baldness. Hair loss associated with this condition is often permanent.

vellus hair: Small hairs found in the scalp that don't grow out to full length or full thickness. Vellus hairs are found inside every follicular unit and make up between 10 to 20 percent of the hair in the healthy follicular unit.

wig: An appliance containing hair that's worn on the head may be used interchangeably with the term "hair replacement system, systems, or hair systems."

Index

• R •

BUSINESS, CAREERS & PERSONAL FINANCE

Accounting For Dummies, 4th Edition*
978-0-470-24600-9

Bookkeeping Workbook For Dummies†
978-0-470-16983-4

Commodities For Dummies
978-0-470-04928-0

Doing Business in China For Dummies
978-0-470-04929-7

E-Mail Marketing For Dummies
978-0-470-19087-6

Job Interviews For Dummies, 3rd Edition*†
978-0-470-17748-8

Personal Finance Workbook For Dummies*†
978-0-470-09933-9

Real Estate License Exams For Dummies
978-0-7645-7623-2

Six Sigma For Dummies
978-0-7645-6798-8

Small Business Kit For Dummies, 2nd Edition*†
978-0-7645-5984-6

Telephone Sales For Dummies
978-0-470-16836-3

BUSINESS PRODUCTIVITY & MICROSOFT OFFICE

Access 2007 For Dummies
978-0-470-03649-5

Excel 2007 For Dummies
978-0-470-03737-9

Office 2007 For Dummies
978-0-470-00923-9

Outlook 2007 For Dummies
978-0-470-03830-7

PowerPoint 2007 For Dummies
978-0-470-04059-1

Project 2007 For Dummies
978-0-470-03651-8

QuickBooks 2008 For Dummies
978-0-470-18470-7

Quicken 2008 For Dummies
978-0-470-17473-9

Salesforce.com For Dummies, 2nd Edition
978-0-470-04893-1

Word 2007 For Dummies
978-0-470-03658-7

EDUCATION, HISTORY, REFERENCE & TEST PREPARATION

African American History For Dummies
978-0-7645-5469-8

Algebra For Dummies
978-0-7645-5325-7

Algebra Workbook For Dummies
978-0-7645-8467-1

Art History For Dummies
978-0-470-09910-0

ASVAB For Dummies, 2nd Edition
978-0-470-10671-6

British Military History For Dummies
978-0-470-03213-8

Calculus For Dummies
978-0-7645-2498-1

Canadian History For Dummies, 2nd Edition
978-0-470-83656-9

Geometry Workbook For Dummies
978-0-471-79940-5

The SAT I For Dummies, 6th Edition
978-0-7645-7193-0

Series 7 Exam For Dummies
978-0-470-09932-2

World History For Dummies
978-0-7645-5242-7

FOOD, GARDEN, HOBBIES & HOME

Bridge For Dummies, 2nd Edition
978-0-471-92426-5

Coin Collecting For Dummies, 2nd Edition
978-0-470-22275-1

Cooking Basics For Dummies, 3rd Edition
978-0-7645-7206-7

Drawing For Dummies
978-0-7645-5476-6

Etiquette For Dummies, 2nd Edition
978-0-470-10672-3

Gardening Basics For Dummies*†
978-0-470-03749-2

Knitting Patterns For Dummies
978-0-470-04556-5

Living Gluten-Free For Dummies†
978-0-471-77383-2

Painting Do-It-Yourself For Dummies
978-0-470-17533-0

HEALTH, SELF HELP, PARENTING & PETS

Anger Management For Dummies
978-0-470-03715-7

Anxiety & Depression Workbook For Dummies
978-0-7645-9793-0

Dieting For Dummies, 2nd Edition
978-0-7645-4149-0

Dog Training For Dummies, 2nd Edition
978-0-7645-8418-3

Horseback Riding For Dummies
978-0-470-09719-9

Infertility For Dummies†
978-0-470-11518-3

Meditation For Dummies with CD-ROM, 2nd Edition
978-0-471-77774-8

Post-Traumatic Stress Disorder For Dummies
978-0-470-04922-8

Puppies For Dummies, 2nd Edition
978-0-470-03717-1

Thyroid For Dummies, 2nd Edition†
978-0-471-78755-6

Type 1 Diabetes For Dummies*†
978-0-470-17811-9

* Separate Canadian edition also available
† Separate U.K. edition also available

Available wherever books are sold. For more information or to order direct: U.S. customers visit www.dummies.com or call 1-877-762-2974.
U.K. customers visit www.wileyeurope.com or call (0)1243 843291. Canadian customers visit www.wiley.ca or call 1-800-567-4797.

INTERNET & DIGITAL MEDIA

AdWords For Dummies
978-0-470-15252-2

Blogging For Dummies, 2nd Edition
978-0-470-23017-6

Digital Photography All-in-One Desk Reference For Dummies, 3rd Edition
978-0-470-03743-0

Digital Photography For Dummies, 5th Edition
978-0-7645-9802-9

Digital SLR Cameras & Photography For Dummies, 2nd Edition
978-0-470-14927-0

eBay Business All-in-One Desk Reference For Dummies
978-0-7645-8438-1

eBay For Dummies, 5th Edition*
978-0-470-04529-9

eBay Listings That Sell For Dummies
978-0-471-78912-3

Facebook For Dummies
978-0-470-26273-3

The Internet For Dummies, 11th Edition
978-0-470-12174-0

Investing Online For Dummies, 5th Edition
978-0-7645-8456-5

iPod & iTunes For Dummies, 5th Edition
978-0-470-17474-6

MySpace For Dummies
978-0-470-09529-4

Podcasting For Dummies
978-0-471-74898-4

Search Engine Optimization For Dummies, 2nd Edition
978-0-471-97998-2

Second Life For Dummies
978-0-470-18025-9

Starting an eBay Business For Dummies, 3rd Edition†
978-0-470-14924-9

GRAPHICS, DESIGN & WEB DEVELOPMENT

Adobe Creative Suite 3 Design Premium All-in-One Desk Reference For Dummies
978-0-470-11724-8

Adobe Web Suite CS3 All-in-One Desk Reference For Dummies
978-0-470-12099-6

AutoCAD 2008 For Dummies
978-0-470-11650-0

Building a Web Site For Dummies, 3rd Edition
978-0-470-14928-7

Creating Web Pages All-in-One Desk Reference For Dummies, 3rd Edition
978-0-470-09629-1

Creating Web Pages For Dummies, 8th Edition
978-0-470-08030-6

Dreamweaver CS3 For Dummies
978-0-470-11490-2

Flash CS3 For Dummies
978-0-470-12100-9

Google SketchUp For Dummies
978-0-470-13744-4

InDesign CS3 For Dummies
978-0-470-11865-8

Photoshop CS3 All-in-One Desk Reference For Dummies
978-0-470-11195-6

Photoshop CS3 For Dummies
978-0-470-11193-2

Photoshop Elements 5 For Dummies
978-0-470-09810-3

SolidWorks For Dummies
978-0-7645-9555-4

Visio 2007 For Dummies
978-0-470-08983-5

Web Design For Dummies, 2nd Edition
978-0-471-78117-2

Web Sites Do-It-Yourself For Dummies
978-0-470-16903-2

Web Stores Do-It-Yourself For Dummies
978-0-470-17443-2

LANGUAGES, RELIGION & SPIRITUALITY

Arabic For Dummies
978-0-471-77270-5

Chinese For Dummies, Audio Set
978-0-470-12766-7

French For Dummies
978-0-7645-5193-2

German For Dummies
978-0-7645-5195-6

Hebrew For Dummies
978-0-7645-5489-6

Ingles Para Dummies
978-0-7645-5427-8

Italian For Dummies, Audio Set
978-0-470-09586-7

Italian Verbs For Dummies
978-0-471-77389-4

Japanese For Dummies
978-0-7645-5429-2

Latin For Dummies
978-0-7645-5431-5

Portuguese For Dummies
978-0-471-78738-9

Russian For Dummies
978-0-471-78001-4

Spanish Phrases For Dummies
978-0-7645-7204-3

Spanish For Dummies
978-0-7645-5194-9

Spanish For Dummies, Audio Set
978-0-470-09585-0

The Bible For Dummies
978-0-7645-5296-0

Catholicism For Dummies
978-0-7645-5391-2

The Historical Jesus For Dummies
978-0-470-16785-4

Islam For Dummies
978-0-7645-5503-9

Spirituality For Dummies, 2nd Edition
978-0-470-19142-2

NETWORKING AND PROGRAMMING

ASP.NET 3.5 For Dummies
978-0-470-19592-5

C# 2008 For Dummies
978-0-470-19109-5

Hacking For Dummies, 2nd Edition
978-0-470-05235-8

Home Networking For Dummies, 4th Edition
978-0-470-11806-1

Java For Dummies, 4th Edition
978-0-470-08716-9

Microsoft® SQL Server™ 2008 All-in-One Desk Reference For Dummies
978-0-470-17954-3

Networking All-in-One Desk Reference For Dummies, 2nd Edition
978-0-7645-9939-2

Networking For Dummies, 8th Edition
978-0-470-05620-2

SharePoint 2007 For Dummies
978-0-470-09941-4

Wireless Home Networking For Dummies, 2nd Edition
978-0-471-74940-0